eye candy

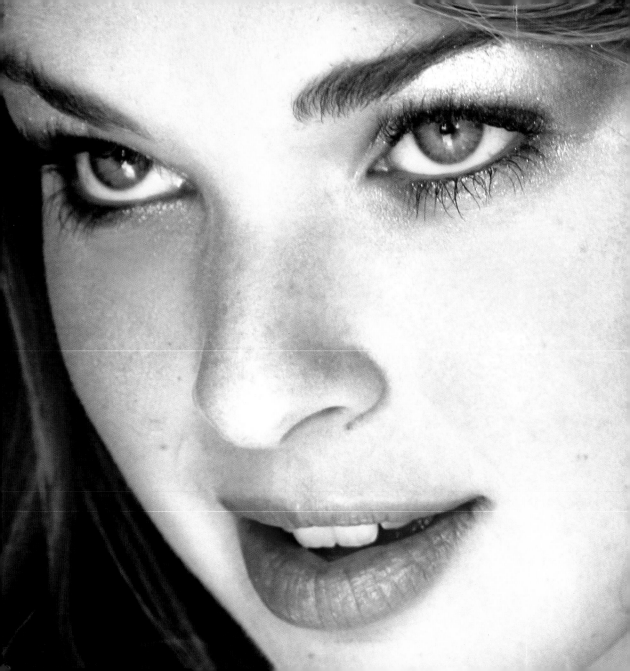

eye candy

55 easy makeup looks for glam lids and luscious lashes

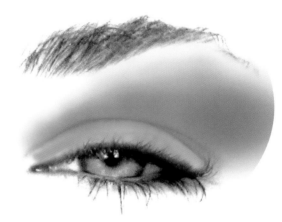

linda mason

WATSON-GUPTILL PUBLICATIONS

NEW YORK

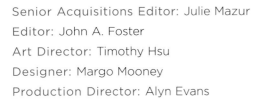

Senior Acquisitions Editor: Julie Mazur

Editor: John A. Foster

Art Director: Timothy Hsu

Designer: Margo Mooney

Production Director: Alyn Evans

Photo on page 11 by Daisy Mason

First published in 2008 by Watson-Guptill Publications,
Nielsen Business Media, a division of The Nielsen Company
770 Broadway, New York, NY 10003
www.watsonguptill.com

Library of Congress Cataloging-in-Publication Data
Mason, Linda, 1946-
   Eye candy : 55 easy makeup looks for glam lids and luscious lashes / by Linda Mason.
      p. cm.
   Includes index.
   ISBN-13: 978-0-8230-9969-6
   ISBN-10: 0-8230-9969-5
 1. Beauty, Personal. 2. Cosmetics. 3. Eye—Care and hygiene. I. Title.
   RA778.M3757 2008
   646.7'26—dc22
                              2007031177

Printed in China

First printing, 2008
1 2 3 4 5 6 7 / 14 13 12 11 10 09 08

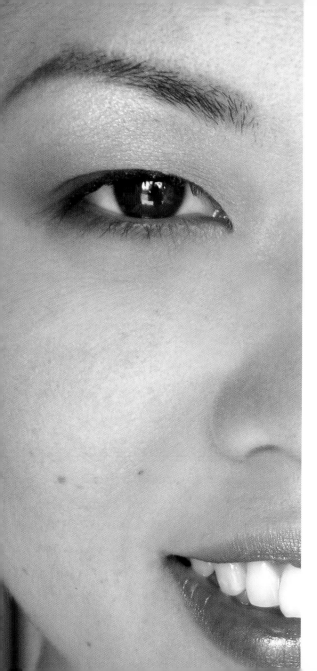

contents

acknowledgments

My life at the Art of Beauty by Linda Mason, in SoHo, New York City, is lots of fun. Many of my clients are passionate about makeup and color, especially eye makeup. They often model for me when I give classes, allowing both my makeup artist students and myself to experiment on them. Therefore, I would like to dedicate this book to my wonderful clients, students, assistants, and interns, many of whom were photographed for this book. I would also like to thank my daughter Daisy, designer Levi Okunov, and hair stylist Almog for always being there for me.

Thank you also to the following models, both professional and amateur (for those who modeled a look, it appears in parentheses next to their name): Akiko (Smooth, X factor); Alana (Midnight, Celestial); Alena, from ID Model Management (Dazzle); Alesia; Alex (Golden); Amy (Neon); Anna (Galaxy Girl); Ashley; Beth (Electric); Candice; Caroline; Charlotte; Chrissy; Coco; Daisy (Bronze Shimmer, Royal, Cleopatra, Sunset); Dani; Danielle; Ellen (Lucky); Isabelle; Jaci (Sophia Loren); Jamila, from Rosario Models (Posh); Jonelli (Spring Fling, Moulin Rouge, Knockout); Julianna (Think Pink); Kate (Sparkle); Katrina (Eye Contact, Warrior); Katherine, from Rosario models; Kristin (Mardi Gras); Lauren; Laurenne, from Click Model Management (Oomph, Firestarter); Lexi (Blue Mood); Lindzay (Casual); Lisa (Playful); Luna (Earth Angel, Dreamy, Audrey Hepburn); Madelyn; Marilinda, from Click Model Management (Coquette); Marisol, from Rosario Models (Mystery, Bejeweled, Mata Hari, Twiggy); Megan; Melinda; Mengley; Ming (Beatnik, Abstraction); Nadia; Nicole B., from Rosario Models (Polished, Colorful, Vanity, Brigitte Bardot, Marilyn Monroe, Mondrian); Nicole L.; Paula (Exotic); Rachel A. (Odyssey); Rachel C.; Rachel S. (Fresh); Rena, from Rosario Models; Rose, from Click Model Management (Glow, Bright Eyes, Me); Saachi; Samantha; Savvy (Zingara); Sanja; Suzanne, from Rosario Models

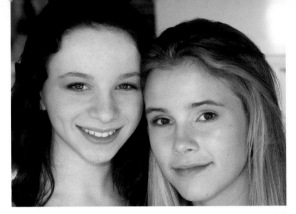

ABOVE: *Taylor (left) is wearing yellow-sand eye shadow with a touch of red-earth in the base of her lashes. See Think Pink on page 81 to acheive Julianna's (right) look.*

(Urban Poet, Asuka Langley Soryu); Talita (Punky); Tania (Soulful); Taylor; Wendy, from Click Model Management. Also, thank you to the following interns and makeup artists and students for creating such great looks: Tama (Posh); Sandy (Earth Angel, Blue Mood, Think Pink, Sophia Loren); Megu (Coquette); Elena Kate (Golden); Kahyang (Spring Fling, Soulful, Smooth); Kelly (Zingara, Odyssey, Midnight, Celestial); Choi (Electric, Moulin Rouge); Ayumi (Beatnick); Tara; Tina (Glow, Bright Eyes, Me); Reiako (Bejeweled, Mata Hari); and Alessandra Grasso (Cream Shadow, Eyelashes).

Thank you to Nancy of Click Model Management, Rosario of Rosario Models, and Darrin of ID. Thanks also to the models who were photographed but did not make it into the book because of space constraints; you were all really great!

Last, but certainly not least, thank you to my agent, Jayne Rockmill, for her help and encouragement, and for contributing such great models; to Julie Mazur, senior acquisitions editor at Watson-Guptill Publications, for giving me another great project, to my very patient and dedicated editor John Foster, to art director Timothy Hsu and production director Alyn Evans, and to Margo Mooney for her fabulous design.

OPPOSITE PAGE, CLOCKWISE FROM TOP LEFT: *My assistant Jonelli; Alex, who also modeled in my book* Teen Makeup; *my assistant Beth; Danielle supporting Rachel during a photo shoot.*

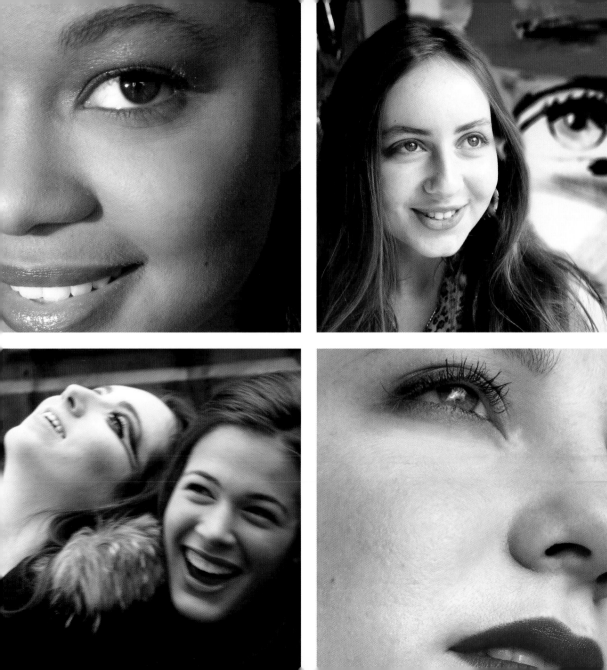

the eyes have it

foreword by Daisy Mason

I had the good fortune to be brought up not only by a world-renowned makeup artist, but one who also happens to be a wonderful, loving mom. Although it might seem, at first, that the two jobs are completely different, the requirements of makeup artist and mom actually overlap quite a bit, as both demand not only compassion but also the ability to recognize beauty and to know how to enhance it.

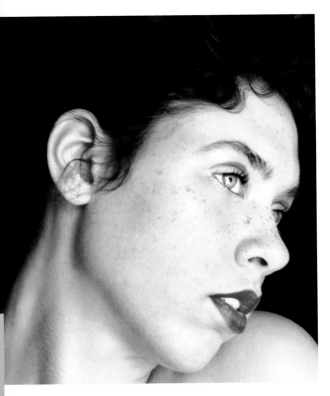

I was born at one of the peaks in my mother's career, when she was working on lots of high-fashion beauty editorials and advertising campaigns. Some of my most vivid, early memories are of accompanying her to the studio and watching her work. I immediately noticed the emphasis that was given to the eyes and how an incredible range of expressions could be created through the use of color and shape. The eyes were often the most time-consuming and detailed part of the makeup process, always being touched up or powdered in place.

As I grew older, I realized how lucky I was to have my own personal makeup artist, and began requesting a "smoky eye" for almost every occasion—I imagined it as my most powerful tool to be treated like an adult. My eyes were transformed into many shapes and forms, depending on the occasion, and were always complimentary and never overwhelming (despite my cries of "More, more!"). Various colors such as turquoise, purple, blue, red, black, gray, and silver were combined and recombined to create countless effects. It gave me confidence to know that the instant I encountered someone, I would leave an impression.

In the past few years, my mom's personal style has shifted and changed (unlike my obsession with smoky eyes.) For a while, bright green eye shadow was her daily war paint, as was bright red eyeliner. Nowadays, it has changed to pale blue shadow and brown-red eyeliner, which is fun and playful with her bright red hair.

Me, wearing bold, sparkly fuchsia and bronze eye shadow for a sunset-inspired look, shown in detail on page 144.

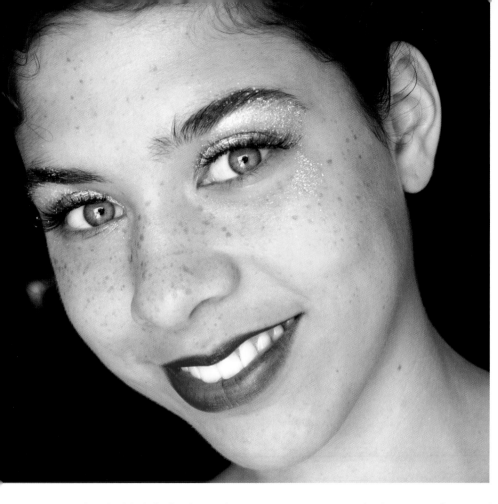

I've lived a life full of color, and it's exciting to see that the beautiful color combinations that my mother has promoted throughout her career are now becoming mainstream, as more and more young people realize how just a little bit of color can enhance their makeup and bring joy to their lives, allowing a safe, bright outlet for all the experimental energy we have.

Whether you prefer neutral shadows or neons, bare lashes or false ones, my mother created this book to help you enhance the two little jewels you use to see the world. I challenge you to explore and enhance your "two windows to the soul" and make them even more powerful and expressive.

—*Daisy Mason, New York City, 2007*

introduction

When I sit a model down to do her makeup, the first thing I am drawn to is her eyes. A new lipstick color can make you feel good, but it is really eye makeup that allows you to transform yourself in amazing ways.

You may have great lips and skin, but everything you do—whether you realize it or not—is directed toward enhancing the eyes. Few know, for example, that the main reason to use foundation to even out skin tone is to eliminate imperfections that might distract from the eyes. Even the decision to skip eye makeup entirely—and just use a strong lip color—greatly enhances the expression of the eyes.

These days, women of all ages feel comfortable wearing eye color, whether as simple accents or dramatic layers of eye shadow. Unfortunately, colorful eye makeup can be intimidating, as it's hard to know where to start or how to create a look or mood. That's where this book comes in. I've included fifty-five eye makeup looks—from simple, everyday looks to glamorous inspirations—complete with directions, tips, techniques, hints, and color palettes to help you find the right colors in your own makeup collection or at any makeup counter. Use these looks to transform your friends, or yourself, and to become comfortable and skilled wearing a daring range of looks.

This book is intended not only as a technical guide, but also as a source for inspiration. When I give makeup lessons, my goal is not to tell someone *exactly* what to do, but rather to stimulate her curiosity, encourage her to experiment on herself and her friends, and to inspire her to enjoy every creative aspect of makeup. I have always been a hands-on person, and I believe the best way to learn is to jump right in and try something. It's only makeup, after all! (Fortunately, I did not become a brain surgeon.) I encourage you to do the same. Try as many of these looks as you can, see what you like and don't like, and change them to suit your own style and coloring. Before you know it, you'll have begun your own journey of self-expression through eye makeup.

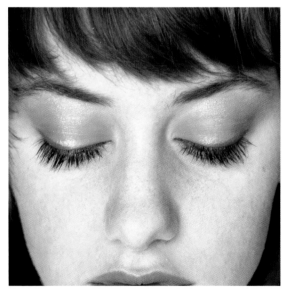

Don't be afraid of color! Experiment with different combinations to create fun and daring looks, like this funky look I call Neon, shown on page 89.

OPPOSITE PAGE: *Me, in front of The Art of Beauty by Linda Mason, my shop and studio in New York City.*

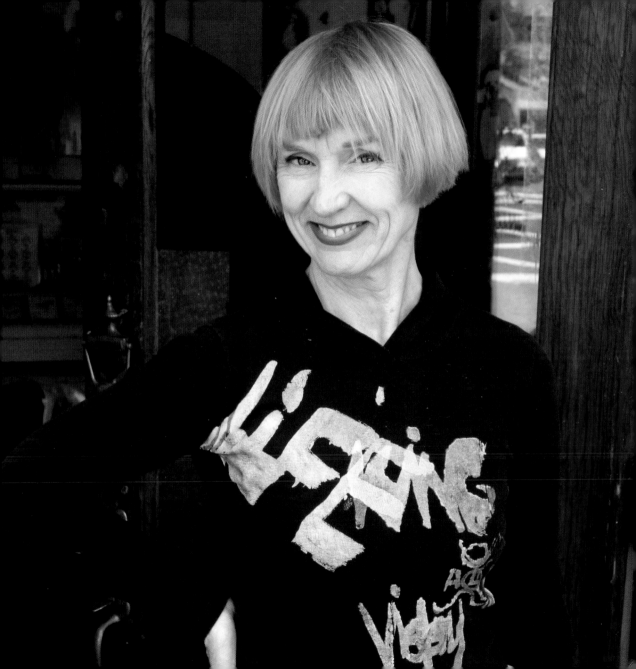

how to use this book

The fifty-five looks in this book have been organized by style, ranging from everyday to flirty, from funky to glamorous. Depending on your personality, you may find yourself drawn to one particular section, or as your mood changes you might like to work your way around the book. Try not to flip past looks that at first glance don't seem like your style. You'll be able to get some pointers from all of the looks—even those that seem the furthest removed from you.

Below, Kahyang applies eye makeup to Tania.

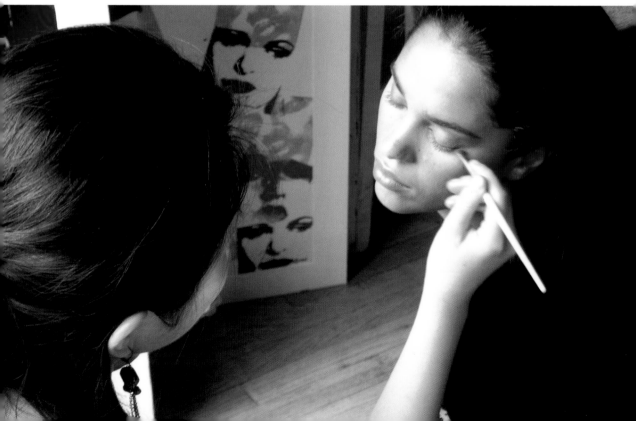

Each look has a list of what you will need, a diagram showing you what to put where, and a palette of shadow colors that you can hold up to your own makeup or use in any cosmetics aisle to find just the right shade.

If you remember these three points, it will make reading the instructions and creating the looks much easier:

1. In each look, the eye shadows are presented in the order in which they are applied. The second color is blended over the first, the third color over the second, and so on—unless otherwise stated.

2. Always press the eye shadow onto the part of the eyelid where you need the most intensity before blending. (This is the reason all the brushes I recommend are fairly firm, as it makes it easier to do this.)

3. Always flick (never rub) the color off your brush *before* dipping it in another color. Only rub brushes that have cream eye shadows or eyeliner on them.

Below are the basic parts of the eye as used throughout the book:

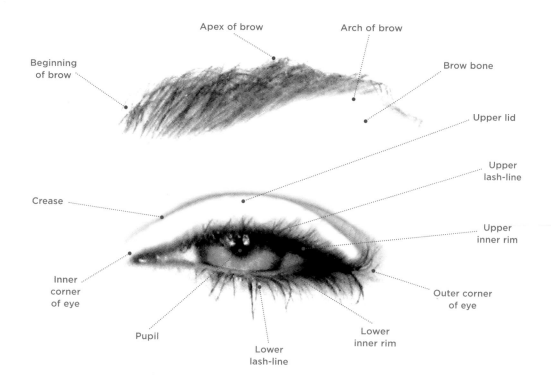

Apex of brow

Arch of brow

Beginning of brow

Brow bone

Upper lid

Upper lash-line

Crease

Upper inner rim

Inner corner of eye

Outer corner of eye

Pupil

Lower inner rim

Lower lash-line

the
basics

In this section I introduce the tools and techniques you'll need to create the looks in this book, as well as how to create your own unique look. You'll learn how to groom your eyebrows and use brow powders, how to apply different kinds of eye shadows with various brushes, how to correctly apply eyeliners, mascara, and flase eyelashes, and the secrets behind making your natural eye shape pop with color and look its best!

eyebrows

Keeping your brows in shape is the foundation to great-looking eyes. The main idea is to keep the area under the brow clean of small hairs, which makes it much easier to apply eye shadow. Even if you prefer to keep your brows natural—which is often the best way to go—there are still fun things you can do to them for those special occasions. The first step to great eyebrows is having the following tools on hand:

A **brow brush and comb** to tame the brows.

An **angled brow brush** to apply brow powder.

Brow pencils and powders to define the brows.

A pair of **tweezers** to clear away stray hairs.

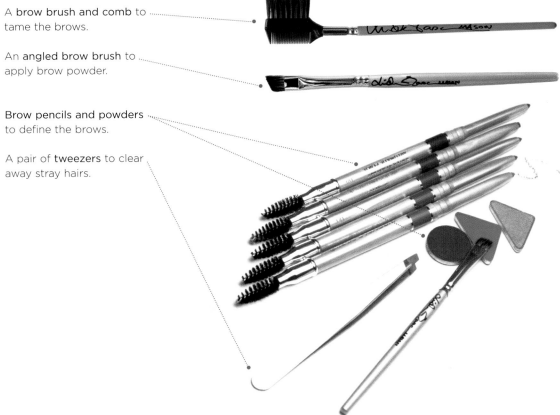

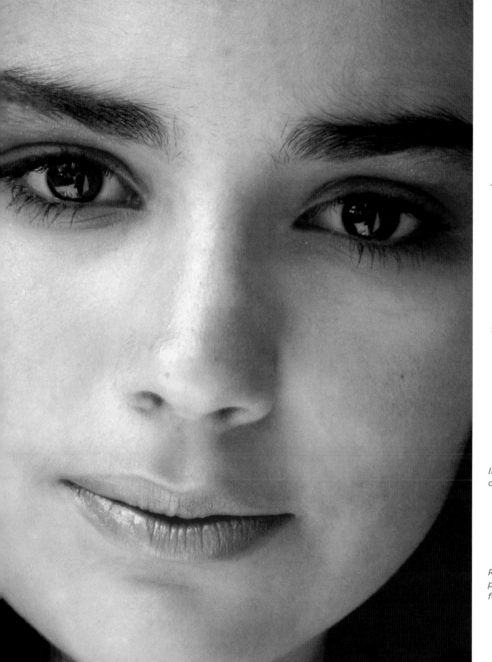

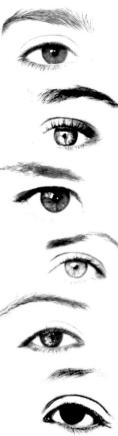

Illustrated above are some common eyebrow shapes.

Rena's natural eyebrows perfectly frame her pretty features.

basic brow care

You may have a great natural brow shape and prefer to keep it that way, or you may want to obtain a natural-looking arched brow. Either way, this section will give you some quick and easy approaches to basic brow care.

If you want to maintain your natural brow shape, you can pluck them with a pair of tweezers at home. Because plucking can be a little painful, choose tweezers with slightly rounded, softer edges. The number one rule when plucking stray hairs is to pluck *only* under the brows. Slip the tweezers under each hair and *always* pull it out in the direction of its growth.

To create a naturally arched brow you'll want to keep your brows thicker at the beginning, gradually narrow them toward the arch, and taper them off at the end.

To find the beginning of the brow, hold a pencil perpendicular to your nose (see **1**). The point where the pencil hits the brow should be the beginning, and all hairs before it need to be plucked. To determine where to start the arch, hold a pencil perpendicular to the outer corner of your eye (see **2**). This is where you should slightly narrow the brow. Now place the pencil at the corner of your nose and angle it up to the outer corner of the eye (see **3**). This is where the brow should end, and any hairs that follow it should be removed.

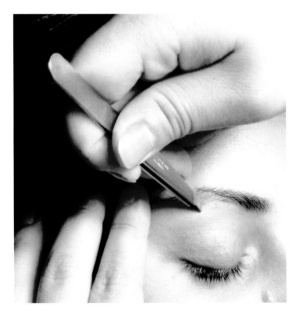

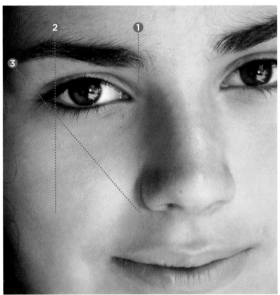

OPPOSITE PAGE: *Tania's lightly groomed brows have a soft, natural look. To obtain this brow, just clean up the stray hairs under the brow.*

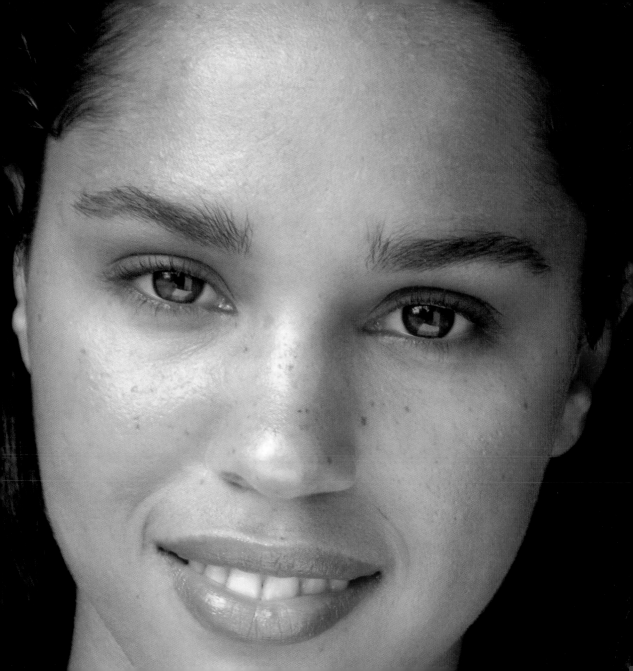

If you have heavy brows, there are a few ways to shape them. The easiest way is to just brush them into shape with brow gel.

You can also thin them with tweezers into a lightly groomed brow. First decide whether you want a straight or a more arched brow, and remember to pluck only *under* the brows and always in the direction of the hair's growth.

Waxing, threading, and cutting your brows will give them a more tailored and sophisticated look, like Sanja's on the next page. However, such techniques are best done by professionals—as experimenting at home often ends with undesired results, like lopsided brows or no brows at all!

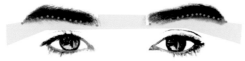

The green sections show where to pluck the hairs for a lightly arched brow if you have heavy brows.

If you have uneven brows, especially at the beginning or arch, strengthen the weaker area of each brow with a brow pencil. Take a blonde brow pencil and fill in the beginning of the brow, using short, sharp strokes. Now, pencil in a little at the arch. Finally, taper the brow off from the arch, taking it down slightly and outward. If you want to give your eyebrows even more of an arch, define the upper part of the brow, especially at the apex. If you have darker coloring, go over the blonde brow pencil with a brunette or black brow pencil.

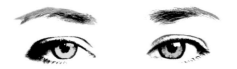

The green pencil shows where to fill in uneven areas.

If you have sparse brows, use an angled brush and brow powder or eye shadow powder to lightly color the skin where the hair is sparse.

If you are a dark blonde, use taupe shadow. Brunettes should use brown shadow. Redheads should start with a blonde brow pencil and then blend in either a red brow pencil or eye shadow (you will have to experiment). For most African Americans, a brunette brow pencil is best—a black brow pencil can look great, but it will look more natural if you start with a brunette color and then work the black brow pencil in.

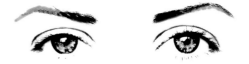

The green pencil shows where to fill in sparse areas.

If you have light-colored brows, or if you're a blonde or redhead and your brows are as light as your skin, you can either leave them alone for a soft, interesting look, or make them more dramatic by brushing taupe eye shadow or brow powder onto your eyebrows with an angled brow brush to darken the hairs.

OPPOSITE PAGE, CLOCKWISE FROM TOP LEFT: *Sanja's tailored brow has a more sophisticated look; by brushing taupe eye shadow onto Lauren's brow with an angled brow brush, her light brow became more pronounced and defined; Wendy's light brows were softly highlighted with taupe shadow and a brow brush; we dramatically transformed Wendy with a painted brow and black wig— who says plucking and shaping are the only ways to create eye-catching brows! Paint a stroke of color over your brows with a paint brush and kyrolan aquacolor, or brush cream eye shadow into the hairs.*

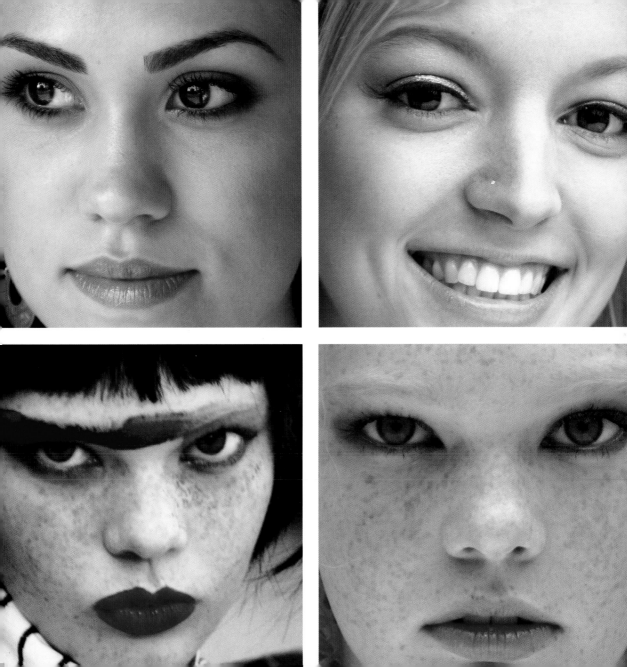

eyelids

Think of your eyelids as blank canvases, ready to be filled with all kinds of color and inspiration. And just as with any type of art, it's a good idea to know the various kinds of materials—and how to apply them—before setting to work.

Eye shadow base and **cream concealer** are applied to your eyes with a fingertip before eye shadow to even out the skin tone of your lid. They produce more accurate eye shadow colors and give eye makeup better staying power, especially when using iridescent shadows. They also make it easier to blend pencil eyeliners, which is helpful if you are creating a strong look with several colors.

Translucent powder can be dusted over lids before applying eye shadow to give colors a softer look. It can also be pressed over your shadows to give them more staying power and to tone them down slightly.

Eye shadows come in matte and irridescent powders, creams, and gels—each in a wide range of colors and textures. (See pages 26-27 for a detailed explanation of each one and how to apply them.)

OPPOSITE PAGE: *Knowing which eye shadows and brushes to use, as well as the different application techniques for each one, is essential for creating mesmerizing looks like this one.*

HINT Unlike the rest of your face, your eyelids have no hair follicles. This means they don't absorb creams like the rest of your skin. Putting moisturizer or eye cream on your lids can cause them to swell and your eye makeup to disappear quickly. Also, if placed too near the lashes, they can irritate the glands at the base of the lashes. It's best to leave your eyelids free of skin creams and moisturizers so your look stays fresh throughout the day.

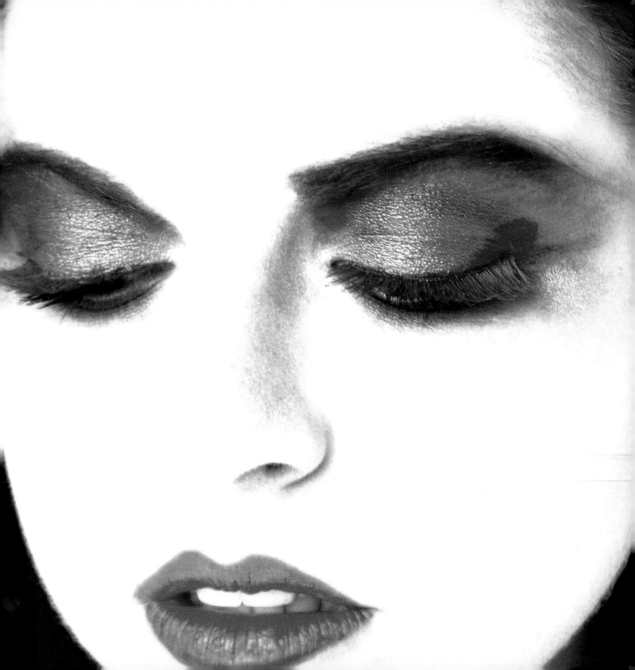

brushing up on brushes

Good brushes will make your eye makeup application swifter and smoother, and are a great investment. Here are the brushes I find the most useful and which are used in the book.

A **blusher brush** is used to give one sweep of color over your lids (or your cheeks).

A **wide eye shadow brush** is great for blending color over the entire lid area. Since it is a firm brush, it should not send flaky eye shadows all over your face.

A **large eye shadow brush** is used to blend or dust eye shadow over larger areas of the lid.

A **synthetic concealer brush** is better (your fingertips are good, too) for cream or gel shadows, as the hairs remain flat when they are wet or greasy.

A **mini blender brush** is tapered and firm, which lets you place delicate amounts of eye shadow into small areas, such as under the eye or in the corners.

A **small eye shadow brush** is used for pressing and blending a highlighter color on top of other shadows. It is also good for blending one color in a specific area.

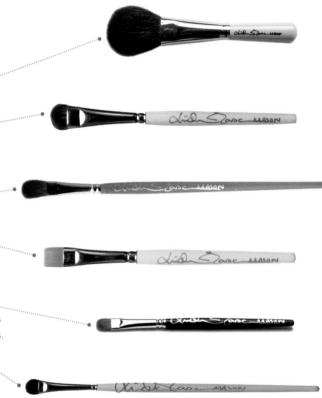

OPPOSITE PAGE: *Lindzay with green, blue, white, and violet irridescent shadows.*

HINT It is extremely important to keep your brushes in good shape and germ free by washing them with soap and hot water. Work the soap into the hairs of the wet brushes with your fingers and then rinse with very hot water. Don't rub them dry; squeeze gently, and then lay them flat. Be sure to let them dry before using them again. A good quality brush, whether synthetic or real, has a lifespan of many years if you care for it properly.

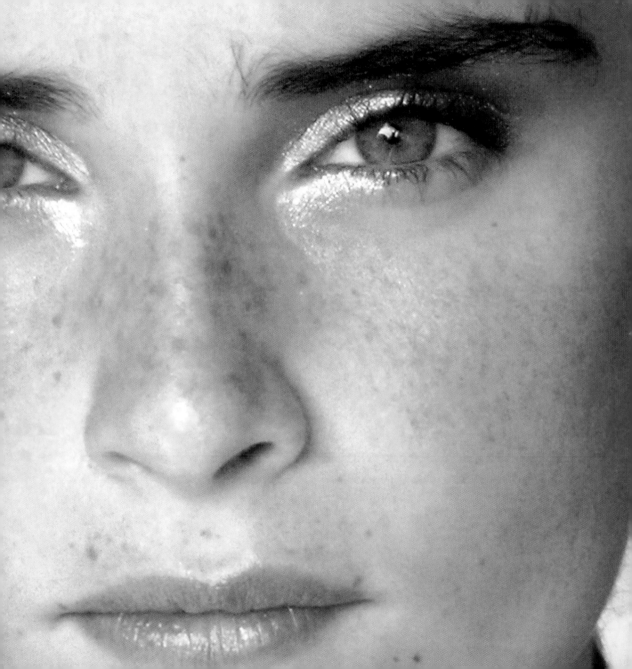

types of shadows and how to apply them

The types of eye shadows and colors available can be totally overwhelming. Only if you are a real pro would I recommend the heavier pigmented shadows that go on with strong coverage. For those of you who prefer a soft, easier look, make sure the eye shadow has a light, transparent feel. You can measure the strength of a color by trying it on your hand or inner arm. When you choose a color and texture, try the different methods of applications explained in this section to see which works best with the product you have purchased.

Powder shadows are the most common type of eye shadow and the easiest to use. *Matte* powder shadows have no shine; *semimatte* shadows have a little shine; and *iridescent,* or *pearl,* shadows have the most shine.

 Matte powders are better for creating depth, enlarging your eyes, and changing their shape, especially darker shades—as they do not reflect light. Use powder shadows delicately, adding little by little to build up color. Matte shadows should always be applied dry. To apply matte shadow, begin by dabbing it on the part of the lid where you want the most depth and strength. Then blend the color outward.

Iridescent and *pearl powders* reflect light, and therefore light up the eye. You cannot, however, get as much depth or enlarge the eye when using them as you can with matte and semimatte shadows. To apply iridescent shadow, dust a light layer over your lid with a large brush, or use a small brush to press it on the lid in one spot for a highlight. Then blend slightly.

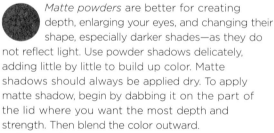 Cream shadows can blend to almost nothing, leaving only a thin film of transparent color. Cream shadows are great, but they don't stay on as well as gel shadows unless you have very large, smooth eyelids. To give cream shadows more staying power, seal them by gently dusting a layer of translucent powder on top. The only downside to this is that it will also tone down the shiny effect that makes cream shadows so special. To apply cream shadow, spread a thin layer over your lid with your fingertip or a synthetic concealer brush.

 Gel shadows can also blend to almost nothing, leaving a thin film of transparent color. They dry more quickly than cream shadows, which means they cannot be as easily manipulated. Gel shadows usually have great staying power. They are applied with your fingertips or a synthetic brush, like creams.

Eye glosses are dabbed on top of your eye makeup with your fingertip for a wet, glossy effect. I love them, but the downside is that you have to make sure that the shadow doesn't crease on the lids.

OPPOSITE PAGE: *You can see the different effects each type of shadow gives. Clockwise from top left, matte powder, iridescent powder, cream shadow, gel shadow, and finally eye gloss.*

HINT Creams are great for blending and strengthening powder eye shadows. Just spread a thin layer of the cream shadow over your lid with a fingertip. Then blend the powder shadow into the cream with a small eye shadow or mini blender brush. If the cream and powder shadows are similar shades, the cream will intensify the color of the powder. If the cream is darker, it will deepen it. Either way, the result will be stronger.

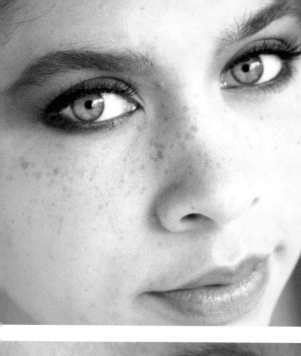
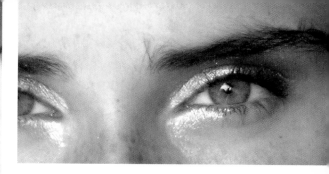
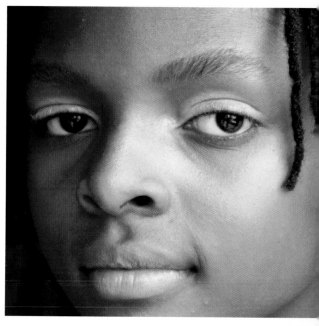
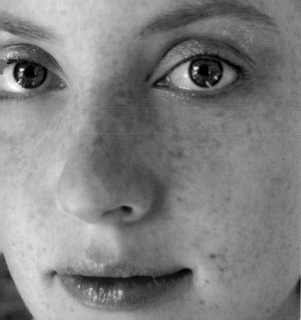
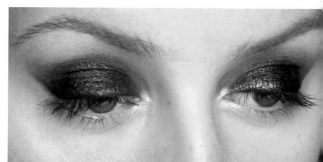

shaping your eyes with shadows

All of us have unique and beautiful eye shapes. Whether your eyes are narrow, almond, large, round, heavy, soulful, small, or inquisitive, eye shadows can be used to dramatically alter the way they look. Here are some tips and tricks to accentuate and alter the shape of your eyes.

To make your eyes look rounder, apply eye shadow or eyeliner starting at the inner corner of the upper lid and going all around the eye with almost the same thickness. You can do this with the crease line, too. Start in the inner corner of the crease and bring it around the outer corner to join the color under the eye.

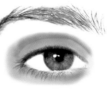

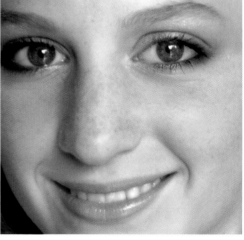

Dark shadow under Coco's eyes make them appear deeper and bigger.

To elongate your eyes, apply a dark eye shadow or eyeliner in the outer corner, along the upper and lower lash-lines. Then use a mini blender brush to blend the color out and up.

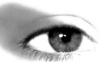

To lift your eyes, blend a deep shade of eye shadow or eyeliner from the outer half of the upper and lower lash-lines, up and out, toward the top of your ear. Be careful not to stop too sharply and create an unnatural-looking line. The color should be blended so that you cannot see where it stops.

To deepen and enlarge your eyes, place a deep eye shadow on the upper lid, from the base of the lashes to the crease, and under the eye.

Eyes with heavy folds, such as Asian eyes, require slightly different techniques to get the same effects. In all of the examples below, you need to extend the shadow from your upper lash-line over the fold. As you do your makeup, open your eye from time to time to see how far you've extended the shadow.

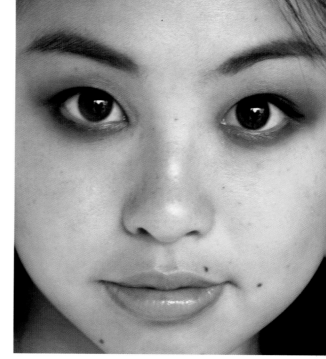

To make an eye with a heavy fold look *rounder,* line the upper and lower lids with eye shadow and then blend the shadow over the fold, making it widest in the center of the lid.

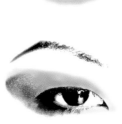

To *elongate* an eye with a heavy fold, blend a deep eye shadow as shown. Don't place the shadow too far up the center of the lid, as this will make your eye look rounder.

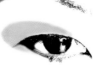

Shadow blended around Mengley's eyes make them appear rounder.

To make an eye with a heavy fold *lift up,* apply a darker eye shadow from the upper lash-line to the outer part of the eye. Keep the shadow much heavier in the upper outer corner and blend it gently outward and upward.

To *deepen* and *enlarge* an eye with a heavy fold, blend a very deep color from the upper lash-line over the fold and underneath the eye. Also, pencil the upper lash-line heavily.

HINT If you want to tone down one of the more dramatic looks in this book, to make it easier to wear in daytime, limit the eye color to the upper lid only, below the crease; do not blend it onto the brow bone or take it into the inner corners.

eyeliners

Eyeliners give strength and definition to your eyes. Lining your eyes with a light color is fresh and fanciful, while a dark color is strong and more sophisticated.

Pencil eyeliners smudge easily and are great for lining the inner rim of the lower eye. You can also use them to get color right into the base of the lashes. And, if you are not quite sure what you are doing and make a mistake, they are easy to rub off.

Liquid eyeliners come in jars, bottles, and tubes, often with a brush. Liquid eyeliner gives you a precise line. It takes a little practice to get the hang of it, so don't get frustrated on your first try.

Cake eyeliners come in pans, like eye shadows. To use them, wet an eyeliner brush and rub it into the cake to make a paste. Then apply the paste to the base of your lashes. Dot the paste into the base of the lashes for a softer, more natural look, or draw a line for a sharper, sophisticated look.

A **white pencil** can be applied to the inner rim of the eyes to enlarge and whiten them.

Gel eyeliners usually come in little jars. They are applied just like cake eyeliners but do not need to be mixed with water, as they are creamy. Gels need to be applied quickly, because they dry fast. They are also waterproof and stay on well.

An **angled brush** is perfect for applying a thicker line to your lid and for smudging.

An **eyeliner brush** has short, tapered, firm hairs that allow you to control the placement and line of your liners.

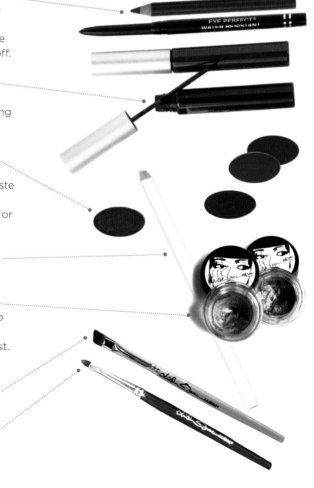

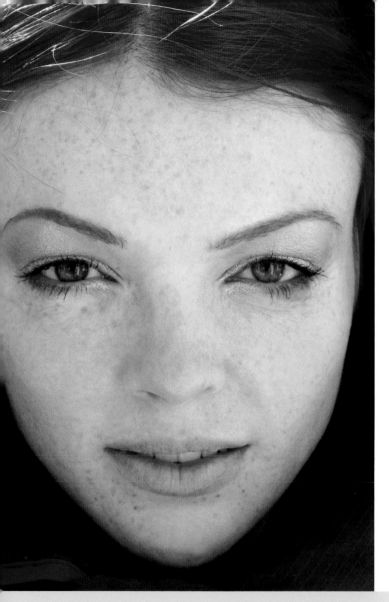

applying eyeliner

To apply any type of eyeliner to your upper lid, begin at the outer corner, as this is where the line should be the thickest. It will also allow you to evaluate how much color you have on your brush (if you are using a liquid, cake, or gel eyeliner) or how heavy the pencil is (if you are using a pencil eyeliner). From the outer corner, bring the eyeliner in and toward the inner corner.

To line your lower lashes, rub the pencil or brush into the base of the outer corner. Then blend inward, keeping the line thinner under the pupil and in the inner corner.

To smudge pencil liner, rub it with either a eyeliner brush or mini blender brush. You can also use a cotton swab.

To achieve a softer effect, use an eyeliner brush to line your eyes with wet iridescent or metallic eye shadow, shown here with silver.

HINT If you have a heavy lid, stretch your lid up with your finger to make sure you apply the eyeliner into the base of the lashes.

eyelashes

As with eyebrows, how you make up your lashes will greatly affect your finished look. When applied correctly, mascara will naturally enhance your eyes' beauty. In this section I will show you some great tips on how to use mascara to make your luscious lashes really stand out!

An **eyelash curler** can give your eye a great lift—just don't overdo it! Over-curled lashes can give you an unflattering, startled look and take away from the natural flow of your eye. When using eyelash curlers, pay close attention to what you are doing and be careful to open the curler *before* pulling it away from your eye. Always curl your lashes *before* applying mascara.

Mascara comes in many colors like blue, green, and violet, which are great for funky, upbeat looks or if you want to soften a strong eye. However, the most popular colors are brown and black. No matter what your hair color, brown mascara tends to look soft and feminine, while black is strong and cool.

Different mascaras have different types of **wands**. Some are curved to shape the eyelashes, coloring the whole lash from base to tip. Others have a denser, deeper spiral, which is designed to hold a lot of mascara for a really thick, heavy application. A wand with shorter hairs that are spaced farther apart is best if you want to separate your lashes while applying mascara at the same time.

A **spiral brow brush** will separate your lashes if they become stuck together after you apply mascara. Wait a few seconds, and then comb the lashes.

For those with lighter colored lashes, use an **eyeliner brush** to paint mascara onto the base of your upper lashes.

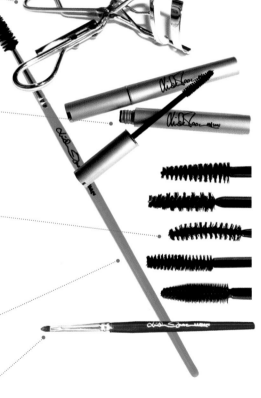

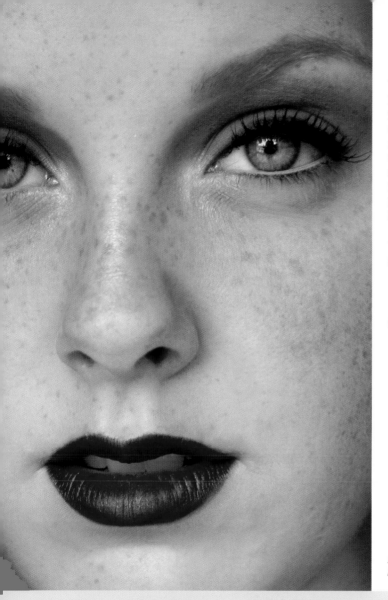

applying mascara

To apply mascara to your upper lashes, place the wand at the root of your lashes. Using a zigzag motion (moving the lashes gently from left to right), sweep the wand from the root to the tips. Starting at the root is especially important for those with light-colored lashes; otherwise, the base of the lashes will stay light and be distracting.

To apply mascara to your lower lashes, point the wand up, as shown below.

When applying mascara to your lower lashes, point the wand up—not in.

Suzanne's strong and defined lashes balance her deep lip color.

HINT If you want a very strong lash, try a two-sided mascara. It has cream on one end, which you apply first, and mascara on the other.

false eyelashes

False eyelashes, or "falsies," are lots of fun and can be a great pick-me-up. They come in so many different shapes and colors—even those of you who *don't* want to be noticed can find the right ones.

Eyelash glue, such as Duo eyelash adhesive (I prefer the white kind, as it dries colorless) holds false eyelashes in place.

Full bands of lashes are entire sets of upper lashes. Bands are better for those with shorter lashes, or anyone who wants the impact of a fabulous band of lashes.

Individual and **cluster lashes** are portions of a full set. These are good if you already have long lashes but want to thicken them.

Tweezers are needed to hold and apply fake eyelashes.

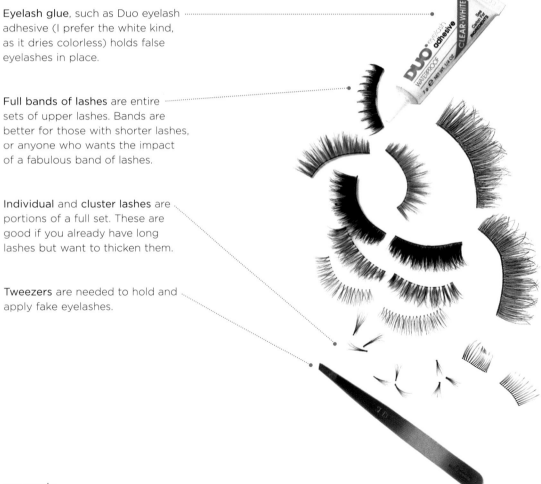

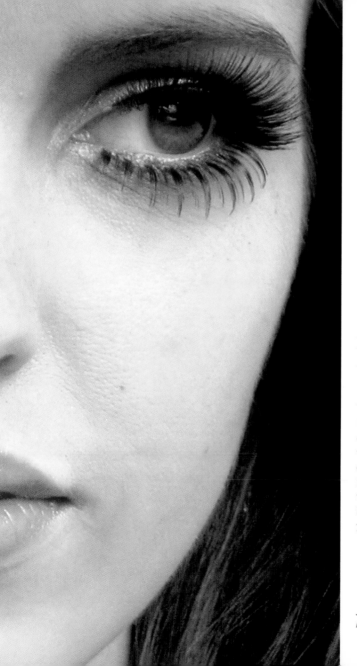

applying false eyelashes

False eyelashes are best applied after the rest of your makeup is completed. If you want a more natural look, use lashes with a light-colored base.

To apply full lashes in a band, apply eyelash glue along your upper lash-line. Wait a few seconds until the glue becomes tacky. Holding the fake eyelashes with tweezers, apply the falsies to the line of glue. Press down on the center of the lash first, then the inner part, and finally the outer end.

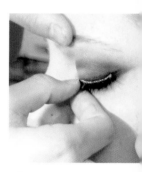

To apply individual lashes, pick up one lash or cluster with tweezers, dip the end of the lashes in glue, and then place them into the base of your own lashes.

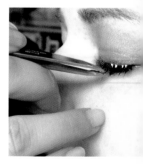

Jamila is wearing full bands of lashes on her upper and lower lids.

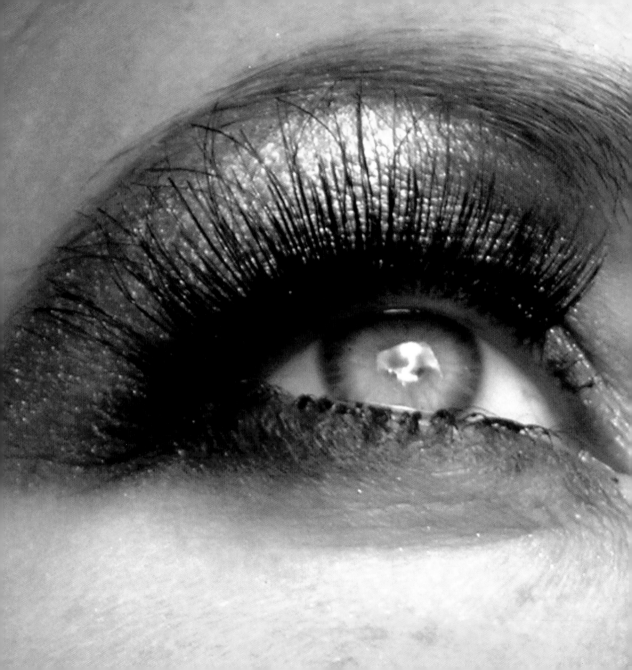

taking it off

Keep your eyes beautiful by gently removing your eye makeup every night. The skin around the eyes is fragile, so take time to find the right eye makeup remover for your skin type. There are many great, inexpensive removers, and they fall into two main categories:

1. Oily removers are best for waterproof mascara and are good if you don't have sensitive eyes (if you do, however, they can irritate them and cause swelling). After using an oily remover, cleanse your entire face with soap or a face cleanser and rinse well to remove all traces.

2. Oil-free liquids or pads are best for sensitive eyes and work well on non-waterproof mascaras. To remove eye makeup, wet a cotton ball or tissue with the remover. Wrap the cotton or tissue around your index finger and start rubbing your lashes from underneath. Then put the cotton or tissue under your eye and close your eye onto it. Now use the cotton or tissue to rub the lashes from above. Once you have removed as much mascara as possible, wipe your lids and brows (wet a new tissue or cotton ball if necessary). Never use dry cotton; always dampen it first. Repeat with the other eye.

If you are wearing false eyelashes, take them off before you remove your makeup so that you can wear them again. Pry the outer corner of the lashes up with your thumbnail. Then hold the end of the lashes with your thumb and index finger and gently pull them off.

LINDA'S TOP 10 TIPS FOR UNFORGETTABLE EYES

1. If your eyes are tired or puffy, lay a cold, wet tea bag on them and relax for ten minutes. Cucumber slices work well, too.

2. If you plan on having photos taken, carry a bottle of eye drops to remove any redness in the eyes—a perfect remedy after late nights of studying.

3. Add some quick gloss to your eyebrows by smoothing petroleum jelly over them with your fingertips. If you want something wilder, try brushing cream eye shadow onto them for a colored brow.

4. When using iridescent or sparkle eye shadows, wait until you have finished and then brush off the shadow that's fallen on your face with your powder brush. Wipe heavier areas with a cotton swab. Don't use your fingertips—it will just blend the shadow further into your skin.

5. If applying eye cream at night, always apply with your ring finger, which gives less pressure.

6. Don't use harsh products near the eyes or rub them strongly.

7. Mascara is not always necessary for a dramatic look. Try leaving it off sometimes!

8. Redness in your eyes may come from eye-strain. Always read with good light and have your eyes checked regularly to see if you have the right glasses.

9. Your health is reflected in your eyes. For bright whites, avoid coffee, alcohol, drugs, or too much time staring at a computer.

10. Smile! It will immediately lift and brighten your eyes.

OPPOSITE PAGE: *Thick and heavy falsies create really dramatic eyes, as well as bronze- or blue-colored falsies.*

everyday

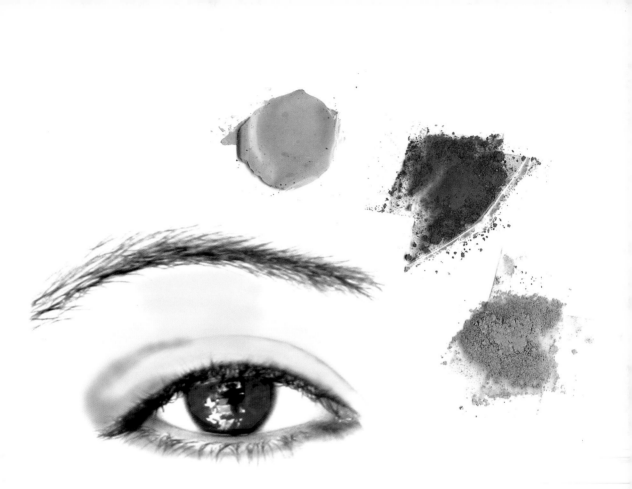

Everyday looks are easy, fast, and discrete. Touches of color—even a hint of glitter—say something about you. As you try these looks, think about what you might add to make each your own. Just remember: this is daytime, so keep everything light. You'll want to stick with only one, two, or maybe three colors.

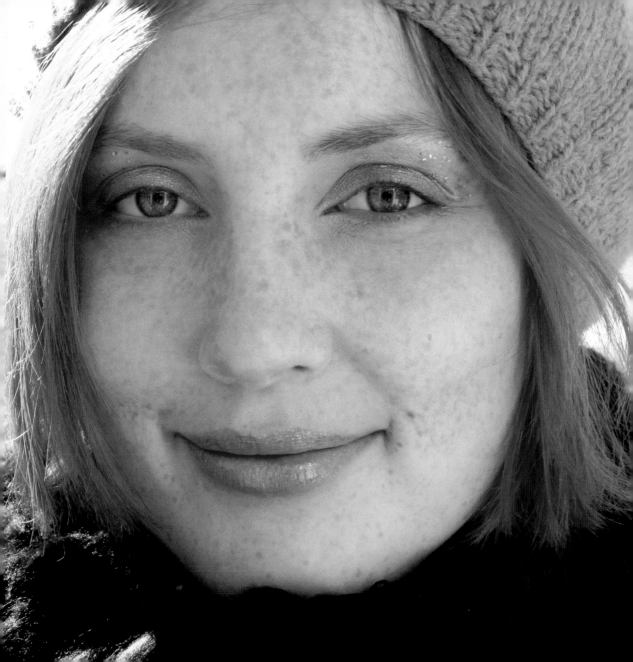

sparkle

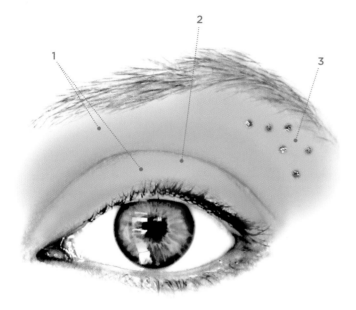

INGREDIENTS

eye shadows
cream metallic bronze
iridescent peach
bronze glitter

other makeup
brown mascara

brushes
synthetic concealer brush
   (optional)
small eye shadow brush

1. Use **fingertip** or **synthetic brush** to blend fine film of metallic bronze over upper lid and brow bone.

2. Use **small brush** to apply peach on upper lid to just past crease.

3. Press a few flecks of glitter into cream on brow bone.

4. Apply **mascara**.

HINT If you don't want to use glitter, press a touch of bright shadow into the cream on the brow bone instead.

We started Kate's look with a very fine liquid base to diminish the slight redness of her skin without hiding her freckles. A peach lip gloss finished the look.

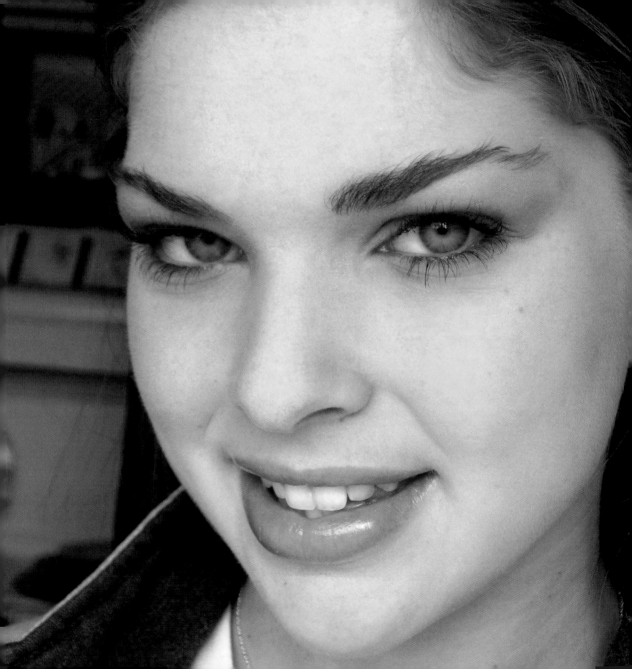

polished

INGREDIENTS

eye shadows
semimatte peach
semimatte taupe

other makeup
black mascara

brushes
wide eye shadow brush
small eye shadow brush

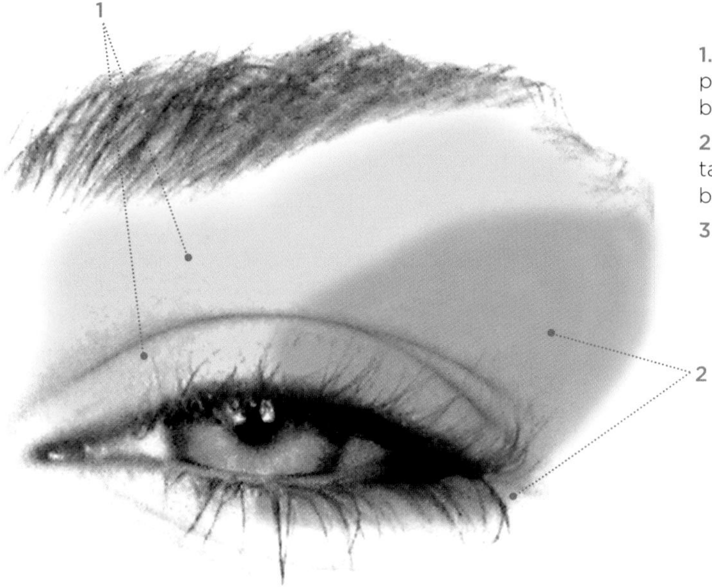

1. Use **wide brush** to apply peach to upper lid and brow bone.

2. Use **small brush** to blend taupe over outer lid area and below eye.

3. Apply **mascara**.

1

2

HINT Try colored eyeliner to strengthen this look for evening.

Nicole's makeup was completed with a soft pink cream blush and pearly pink lip gloss.

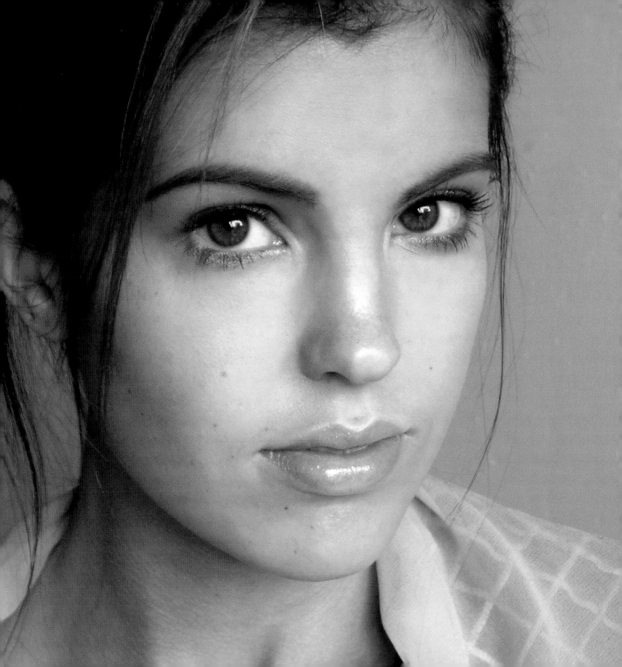

posh

INGREDIENTS

eye shadows
iridescent green
matte brown
iridescent gold

other makeup
black mascara

brushes
eyeliner brush
mini blender brush

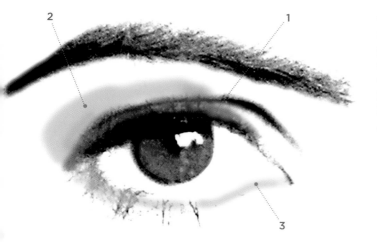

1. Use **eyeliner brush** to line upper lid with green.

2. Use **mini blender brush** to apply brown just above crease.

3. Use **eyeliner brush** to line lower lid with gold.

4. Apply **mascara**.

HINT If you have light-colored lashes, rub dark green pencil eyeliner into the base of your upper lashes to make your eyes pop.

We finished Jamila's look with coral blush and coral lipstick topped with yellow lip gloss.

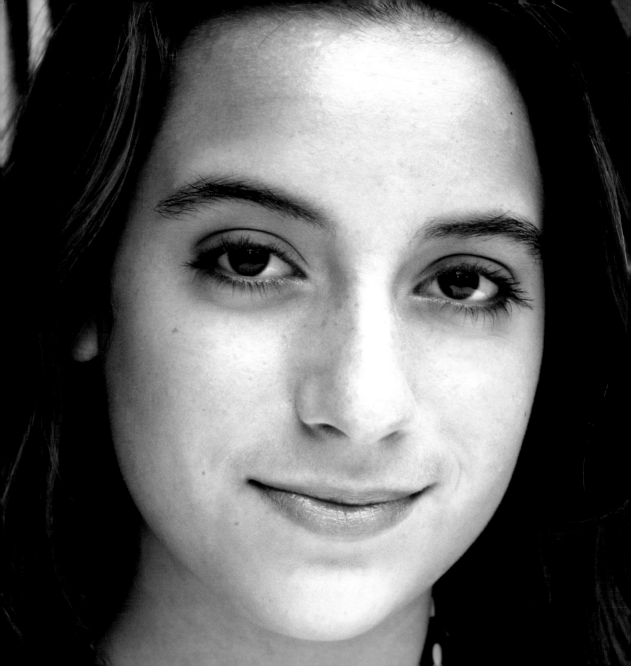

earth
angel

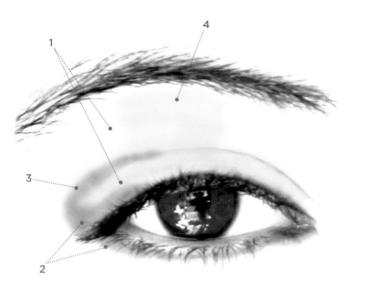

INGREDIENTS

eye shadows
cream lilac
matte violet
semimatte peach

other makeup
black mascara

brushes
synthetic concealer brush
   (optional)
eyeliner brush
mini blender brush
small eye shadow brush

1. Use **fingertips** or **synthetic brush** to blend lilac on upper lid and brow bone.

2. Use **eyeliner brush** to apply violet to outer corner of upper lash-line and under eye.

3. Use **mini blender brush** to blend violet onto outer half of crease.

4. Use **small brush** to highlight center of eye with peach.

5. Apply **mascara**.

HINT Finish with a layer of iridescent yellow shadow to transform this into a soft evening look.

To complete Luna's look, we used coral blush and soft pearly pink lip gloss.

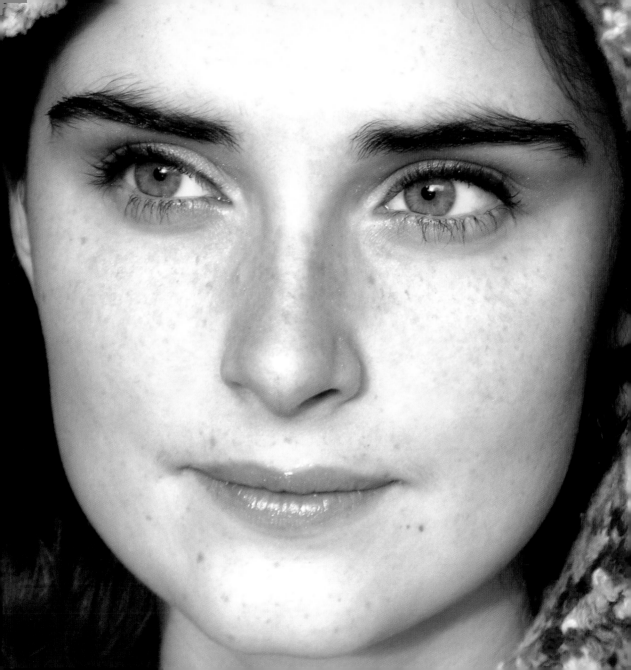

casual

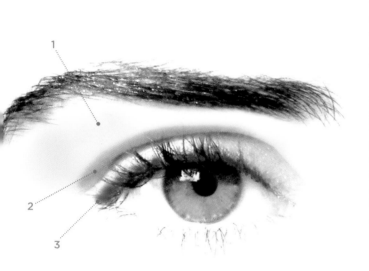

INGREDIENTS

eye shadows
semimatte peach
matte reddish-brown

other makeup
reddish-brown cake or
    liquid eyeliner
black mascara

brushes
wide eye shadow brush
mini blender brush
eyeliner brush

1. Use **wide brush** to apply peach over upper lid and brow bone.

2. Use **mini blender brush** to define crease with reddish-brown.

3. Use **eyeliner brush** to apply delicate line of eyeliner along upper lash-line.

4. Apply **mascara**.

HINT Lindzay's fresh pink coloring didn't need blush. If your skin is less rosy, add blush to the apples of your cheeks.

We completed Lindzay's look with berry lip gloss.

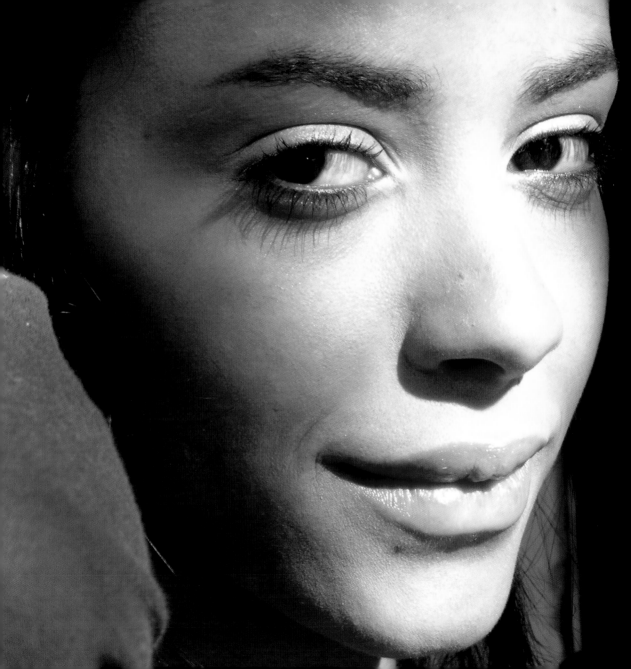

coquette

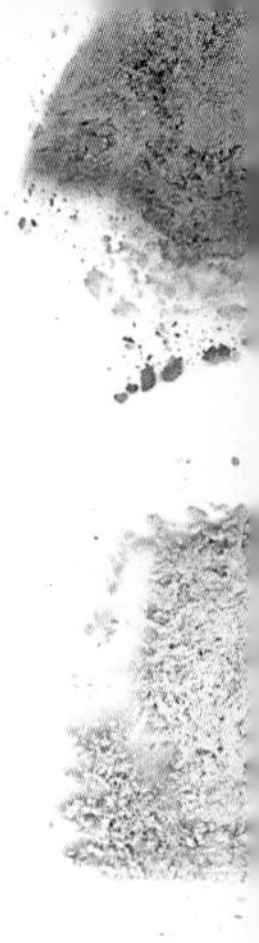

INGREDIENTS

eye shadows
semimatte taupe
iridescent pale lilac

other makeup
black mascara

brushes
small eye shadow brush
mini blender brush

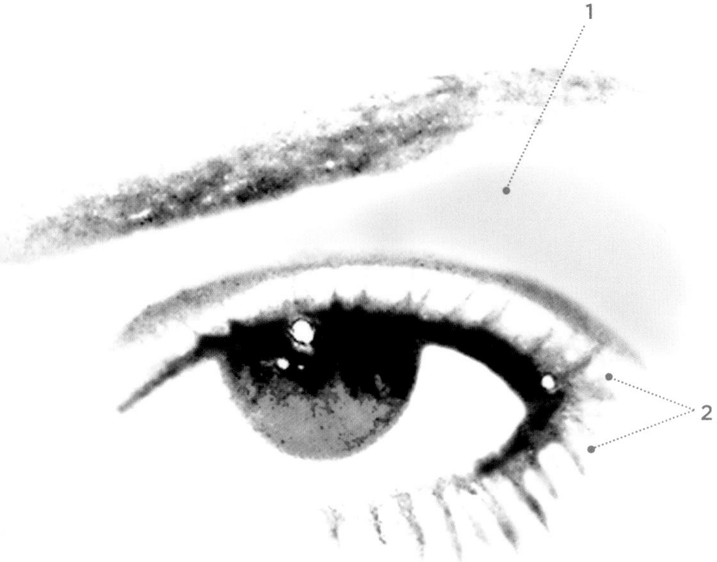

1. Use **small brush** to apply taupe from just above crease to brow bone.

2. Wet **mini blender brush** with pale lilac and line upper and lower lids.

3. Apply **mascara**.

1

2

HINT This eye goes well with a strong, red lip color.

Marilinda's look includes a reddish-brown cream blush and clear lip gloss.

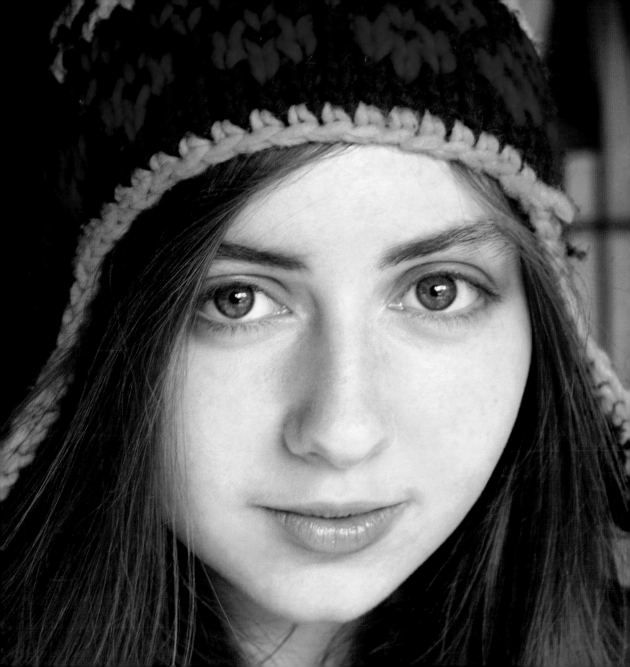

golden

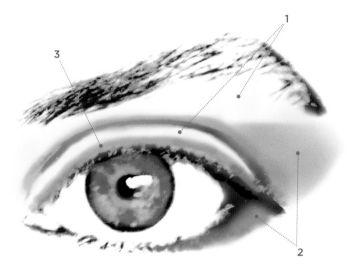

INGREDIENTS

eye shadows
matte ivory
iridescent peach bronze
cream mustard

other makeup
brown mascara

brushes
large eye shadow brush
small eye shadow brush
eyeliner brush

1. Use large brush to cover upper lid and brow bone with ivory.

2. Use small brush to apply bronze below eye and into crease, blending out.

3. Use eyeliner brush to line upper lid with mustard.

4. Apply mascara.

HINT Use your finger to add a dot of clear lip gloss over the makeup on each lid to create a wet look.

Alex's makeup was completed with reddish-brown cream blush and yellow lip gloss.

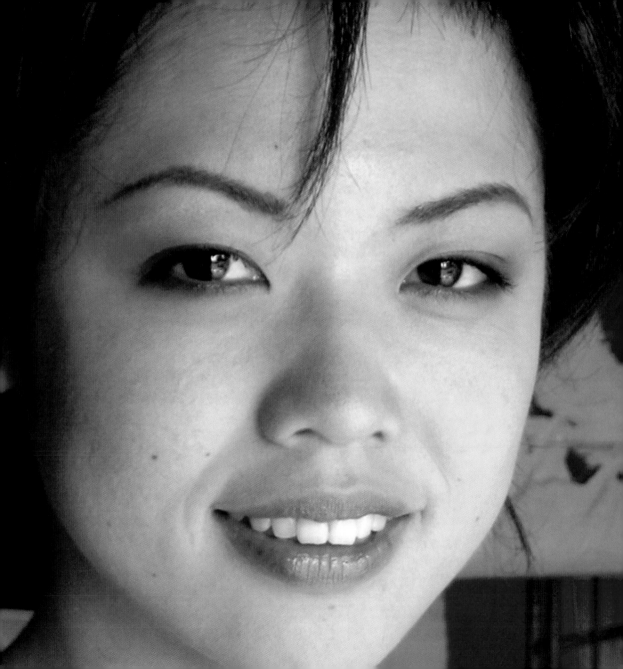

smooth

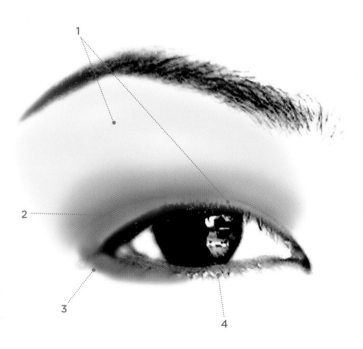

INGREDIENTS

eye shadows
semimatte peach
matte reddish-brown

other makeup
black mascara
brown pencil eyeliner

brushes
large eye shadow brush
small eye shadow brush

1. Use **large brush** to apply peach to upper lid and brow bone.

2. Use **small brush** to apply reddish-brown on upper lid from lash-line to past crease, blending so that it tapers into the peach.

3. Use **small brush** to apply reddish-brown under lower lash-line.

4. Apply **eyeliner** to inner rim.

5. Apply **mascara**.

HINT Line your upper lid with black eyeliner for extra strength.

We finished Akiko's makeup with reddish-brown cream blush and red lip stain.

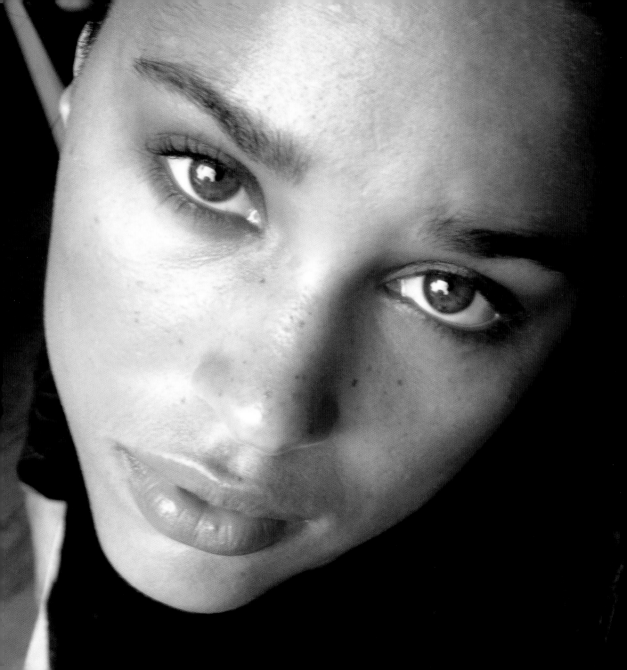

soulful

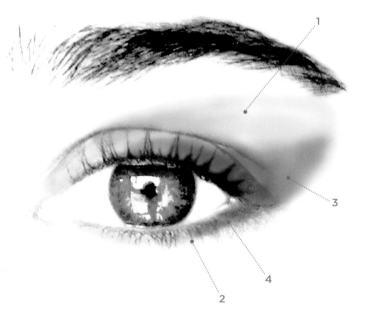

INGREDIENTS

eye shadows
matte stone
matte dark gray

other makeup
black mascara

brushes
small eye shadow brush
mini blender brush

1. Use **small brush** to apply stone to upper lid, blending from base of lashes and going out and up, as shown.

2. Use **mini blender brush** to line lower eye with stone.

3. Layer dark gray on outer part of upper lid with **mini blender brush** from base of lashes, winging out.

4. Use **mini blender brush** to line lower eye with dark gray.

5. Apply **mascara**.

HINT Finish by adding a touch of metallic silver shadow to the center of each lid to add sparkle and light.

Tania's look was completed with reddish-brown cream blush and coral lipstick.

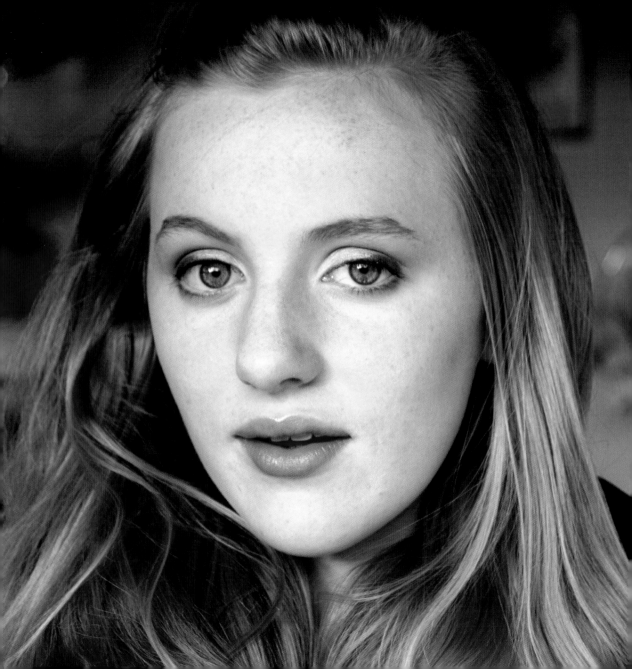

lucky

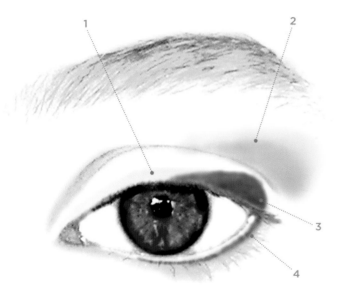

INGREDIENTS

eye shadows
iridescent pale green
semimatte acid green
matte deep green

other makeup
dark gray pencil eyeliner
black mascara

brushes
eyeliner brush
small eye shadow brush
mini blender brush

1. Use **eyeliner brush** to line upper lid with pale green.

2. Use **small brush** to apply acid green in crease and just above it.

3. Use **eyeliner brush** to create shape with deep green on upper lid, as shown.

4. Line outer corner of lower lid with eyeliner and then smudge with **mini blender brush**.

5. Apply **mascara**.

HINT These colors stand out best on paler skins.

We completed Ellen's look with soft pink cream blush and a light touch of orange lipstick covered with yellow gloss.

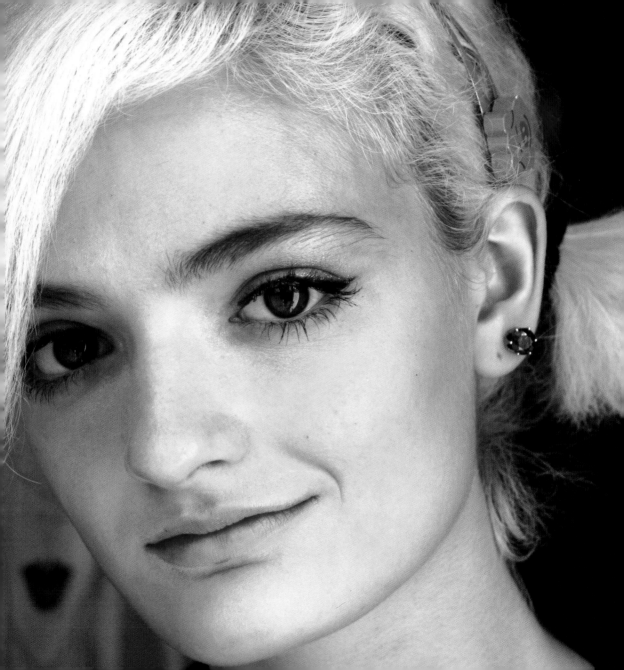

punky

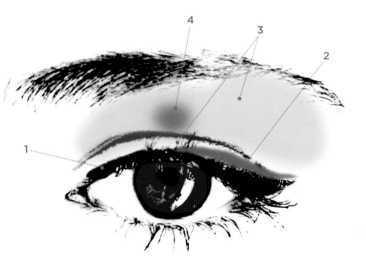

INGREDIENTS

eye shadows
iridescent aqua
iridescent beige
iridescent pink

other makeup
black cake or pencil eyeliner
black mascara

brushes
eyeliner brush
large eye shadow brush
mini blender brush

1. Line upper lash-line with **black eyeliner**, keeping the line narrow over pupil, thicker in outer corner, and extending it a little past eye.

2. Make sure **eyeliner brush** is free of eyeliner and then use it to draw an aqua line above the black one in the outer corner.

3. Use **large brush** to lightly dust beige over upper lid and brow bone.

4. Use **mini blender brush** to press a touch of pink at center of eye, just above crease.

5. Apply **mascara**.

HINT To transform this look into a more formal one, apply aqua shadow under the eyes.

Talitha's look was finished with soft pink blush and clear lip gloss.

flirtatious

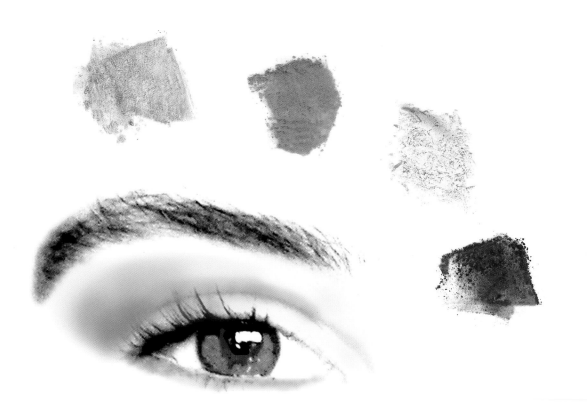

Flirtatious looks are soft and colorful, fun and light-hearted. They are your heart on a warm spring day. The looks in this section are inspired by romantic color combinations, such as pink and blue, or pink and green with violet highlights.

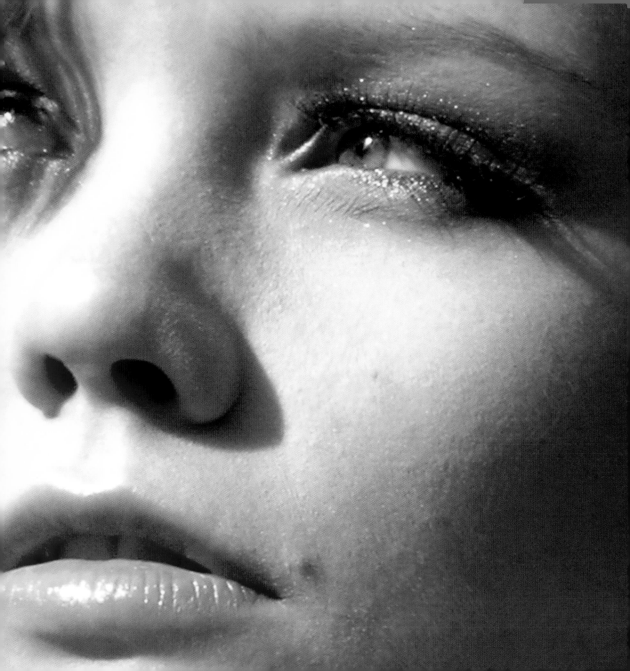

dazzle

INGREDIENTS

eye shadows
iridescent teal
iridescent gold

other makeup
black mascara

brushes
small eye shadow brush
mini blender brush

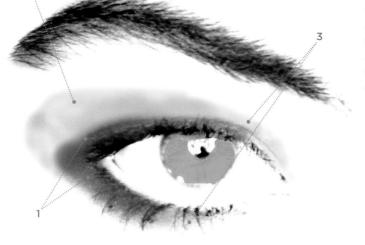

1. Use **mini blender brush** to line upper and lower lids with teal.

2. Use **mini blender brush** to apply gold in crease, blending out.

3. Use **small brush** to apply gold to inner corners of eye.

4. Apply **mascara**.

HINT Blend the gold just over the crease, not all the way up to the brow.

Alena's look was finished with soft pink cream blush and coral lipstick.

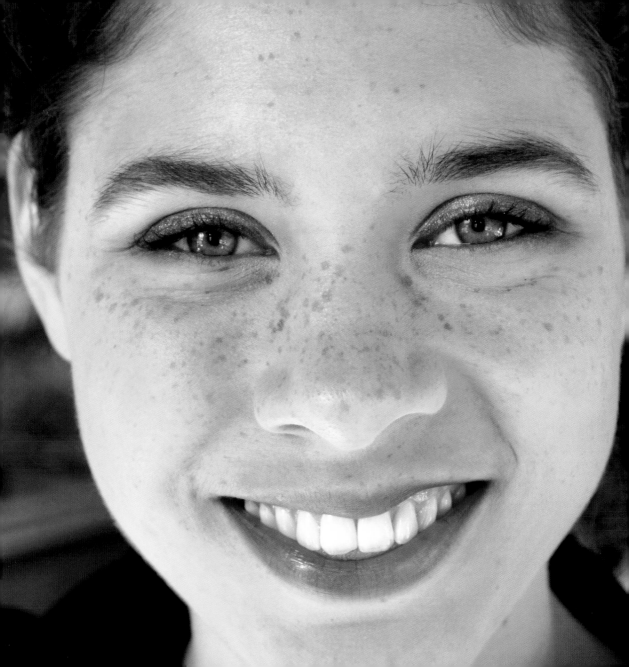

bronze shimmer

INGREDIENTS

eye shadows
iridescent pale lilac
semimatte taupe

other makeup
bronze gel eyeliner
gray pencil eyeliner
black mascara

brushes
mini blender brush
eyeliner brush

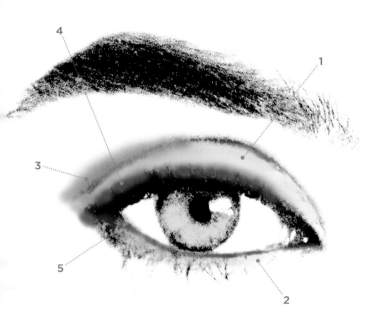

1. Use **mini blender brush** to cover upper lid with pale lilac, from lash-line to crease.

2. Use **eyeliner brush** to line lower lid with pale lilac.

3. Use **mini blender brush** to blend taupe into outer half of crease.

4. Line upper lid with **bronze gel eyeliner**.

5. Line inner rim of lower lid with **gray pencil eyeliner**.

6. Apply **mascara**.

HINT For darker eyes, blend taupe over the entire lid instead and add a touch of pale lilac over the brow as a highlight.

Daisy's makeup includes reddish-brown cream blush and brown lipstick.

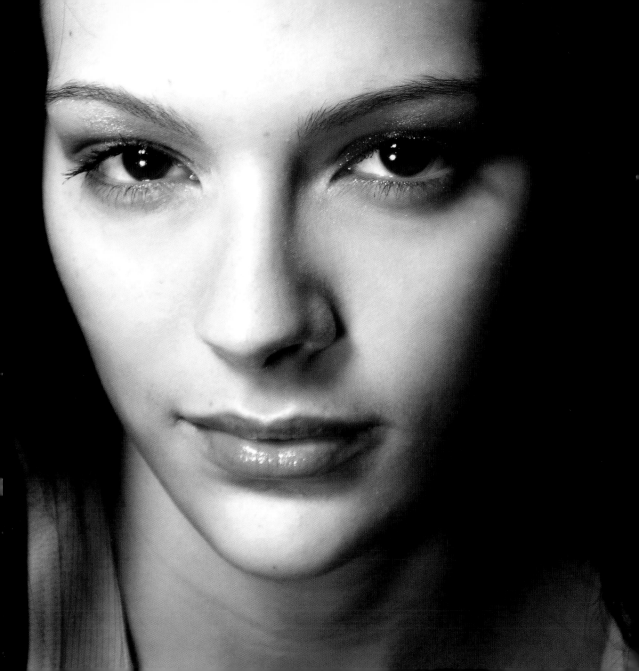

mystery

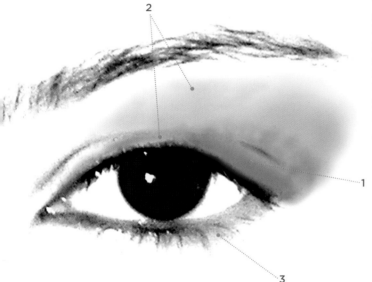

eye shadows
iridescent sparkly fuchsia
iridescent silver

other makeup
black mascara

brushes
small eye shadow brush
mini blender brush

1. Use **small brush** to apply sparkly fuchsia along upper lash-line and blend outward.

2. Use **mini blender brush** to apply silver next to sparkly fuchsia in center of lid and under brow bone.

3. Use **mini blender brush** to line lower lid with silver.

4. Apply **mascara**.

HINT To soften this look, don't place color on the inner corners of the eye or on the brow bone.

Reddish-brown cream blush and clear lip gloss was used to complete Marisol's look.

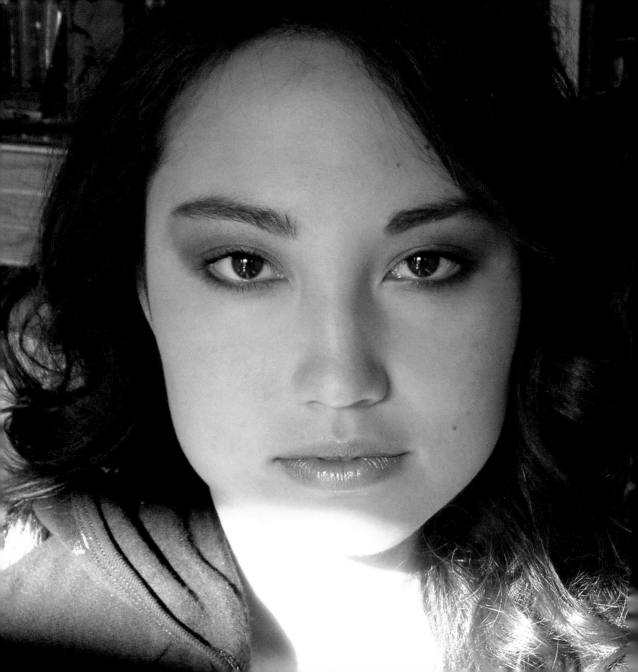

eye
contact

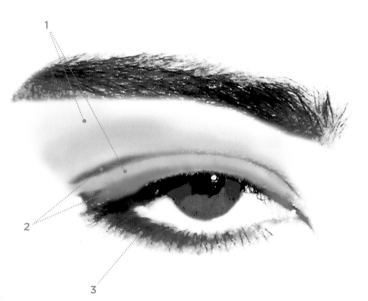

INGREDIENTS

eye shadows
iridescent olive
iridescent bright green
matte burgundy-red

other makeup
black mascara

brushes
wide eye shadow brush
mini blender brush
eyeliner brush

1. Use **wide brush** to cover upper lid with olive, blending it up and out and tapering off at brow bone.

2. Use **mini blender brush** to line upper lid and crease with bright green.

3. Use **eyeliner brush** to line lower lid with burgundy-red.

4. Apply **mascara**.

HINT If you want to give an upward lift to your eyes, add a dot of navy blue shadow to the outer corner of the upper lash-line.

To finish Katrina's look, we added coral blush and soft pearly pink lip gloss.

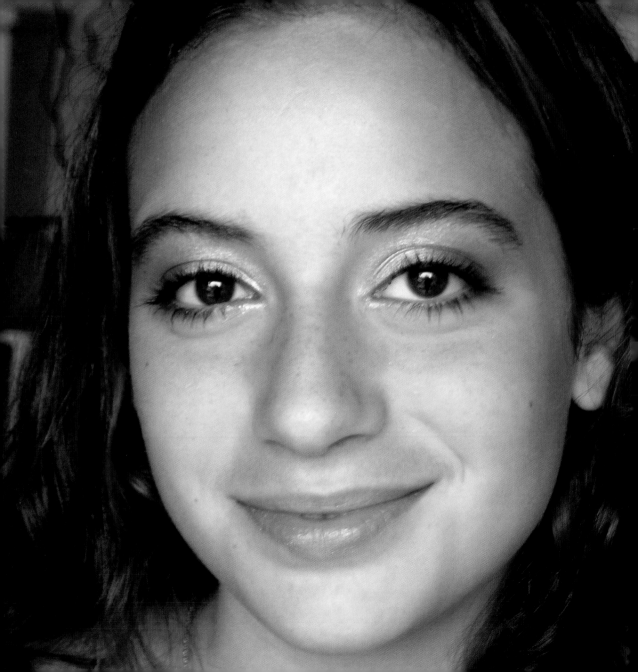

dreamy

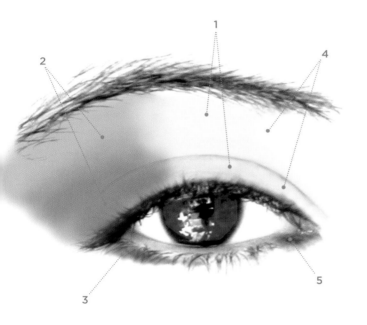

INGREDIENTS

eye shadows
cream iridescent pale green
iridescent dark-gold
metallic silver

other makeup
black mascara

brushes
small eye shadow brush
mini blender brush
eyeliner brush

1. Use your **fingertip** to apply thin layer of pale green over upper lid and brow bone.

2. Use **small brush** to blend dark-gold over half of upper lid and brow bone.

3. Use **mini blender brush** to line outer half of lower lid with dark-gold.

4. Use **small brush** to apply silver to inner half of upper lid and brow bone, blending it into the dark-gold with no separation.

5. Use **eyeliner brush** to apply silver to inner corner of lower lid.

6. Apply **mascara**.

HINT You might find this look easier to wear if you don't take the silver all the way to the inner corners of your eye or under your brow.

We finished Luna's look with reddish-brown cream blush and berry lip gloss.

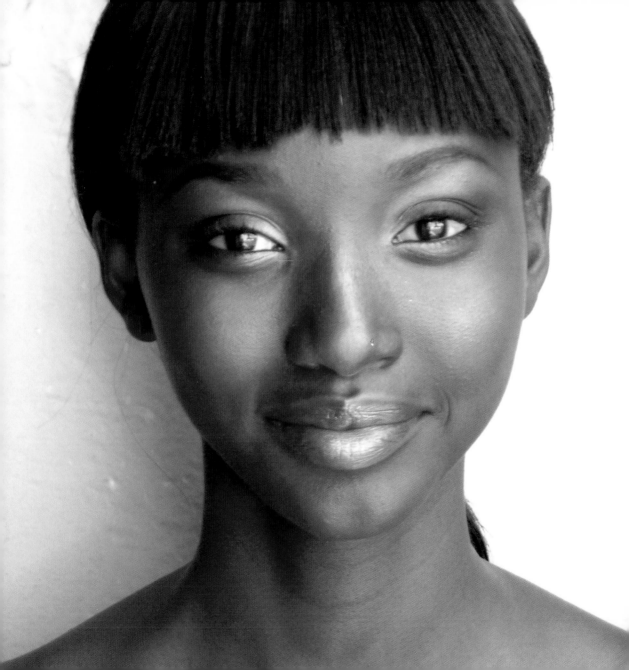

glow

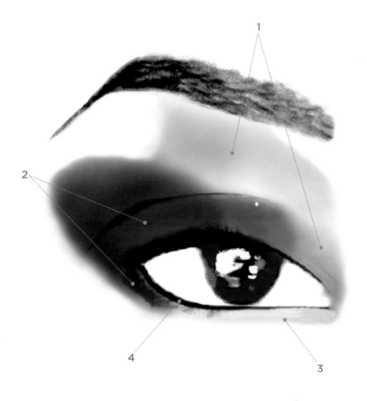

INGREDIENTS

eye shadows
iridescent gold
matte black

other makeup
black pencil eyeliner
black mascara

brushes
large eye shadow brush
mini blender brush

1. Use **large brush** to blend gold over inner half of upper lid and brow bone.

2. Use **mini blender brush** to apply black over upper lid to crease, overlapping the gold. Blend black up and out, putting a little under the outer corner of eye as well.

3. Use **mini blender brush** to line inner half of lower lid with gold.

4. Line inner rim of lower eye with **eyeliner**.

5. Apply **mascara**.

HINT Dust a little gold shadow on your lips for a soft highlight.

Rose's look was completed with reddish-brown cream blush and yellow lip gloss topped with a touch of gold.

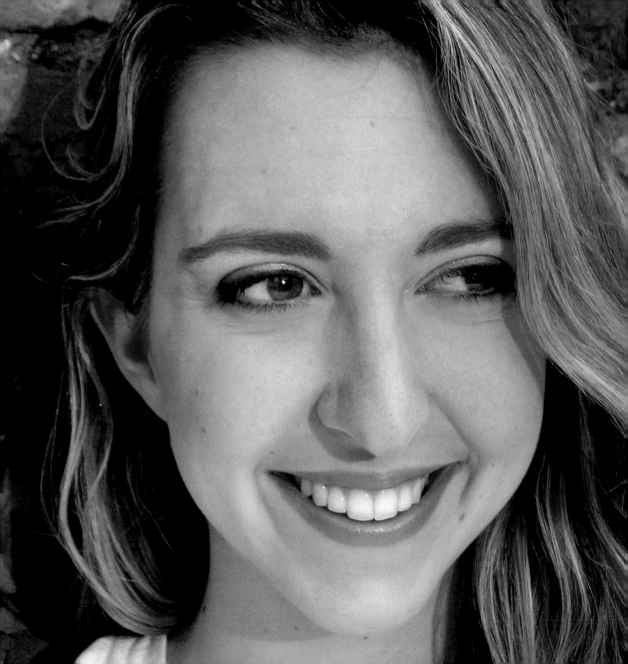

fresh

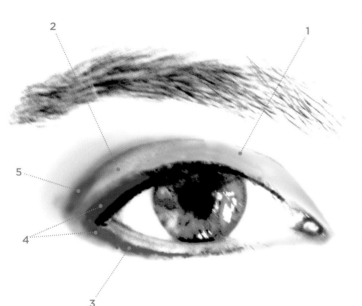

INGREDIENTS

eye shadows
iridescent green-gold
matte violet
matte dark purple

other makeup
black mascara

brushes
small eye shadow brush
eyeliner brush
mini blender brush

1. Use **small brush** to apply green-gold to inner two-thirds of upper lid, up to crease.

2. Use **small brush** to apply violet from outer third of lid to crease.

3. Use **small brush** to line lower lid with violet.

4. Use **eyeliner brush** to apply purple along outer corners of upper and lower lash-lines.

5. Use **mini blender brush** to strengthen crease with a touch of purple.

6. Apply **mascara**.

HINT For an extra lift, add a touch of black pencil eyeliner to the outer corner of the upper lid.

We finished Rachel's look with rose blush and pink lipstick.

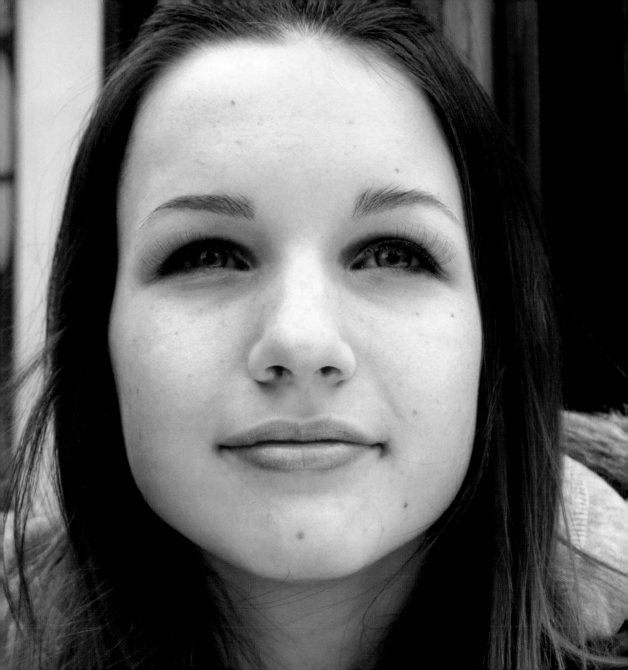

galaxy girl

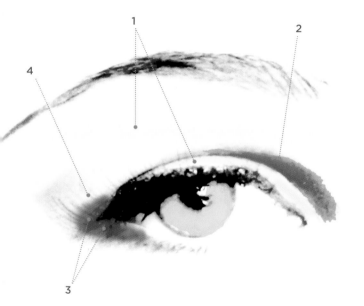

INGREDIENTS

eye shadows
semimatte light blue
matte violet
matte khaki

other makeup
brown mascara
brown false eyelashes

brushes
wide eye shadow brush
mini blender brush
eyeliner brush (optional)

1. Use **wide brush** to apply light blue over upper lid and brow bone.

2. Use **mini blender brush** to accentuate inner half of crease with violet.

3. Use **mini blender brush** or **eyeliner brush** to accentuate outer corner of eye with khaki.

4. Apply lots of **mascara** and long, light **falsies**.

HINT   If you have deep or closely set eyes, apply the violet to the *center* of your crease, not the inner corner.

We completed Anna's look with iridescent pink lip gloss.

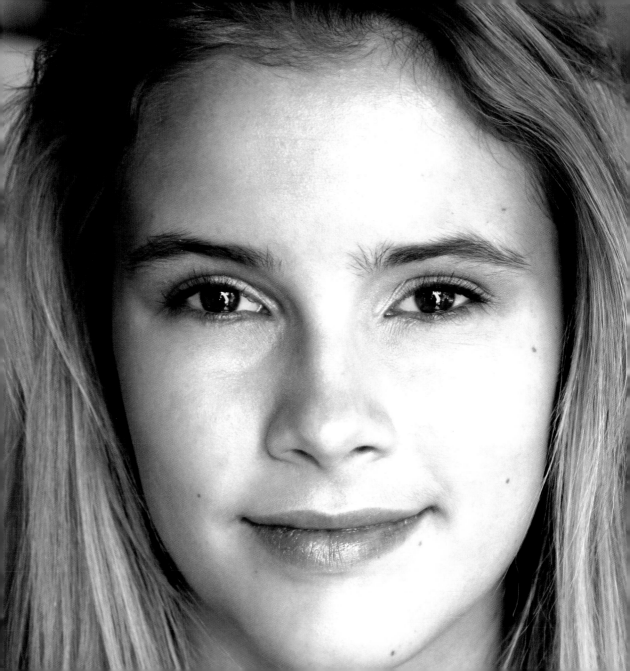

think pink

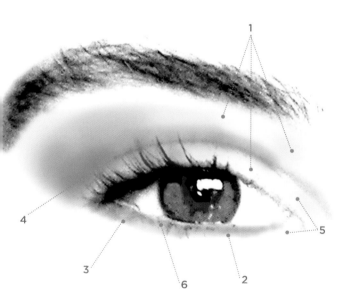

INGREDIENTS

eye shadows
iridescent pink
matte sparkly fuchsia
iridescent pearl
iridescent lapis blue

other makeup
black mascara

brushes
wide eye shadow brush
small eye shadow brush
mini blender brush
eyeliner brush

1. Use **wide brush** to sweep pink over upper lid and brow bone.

2. Use **wide brush** to line lower inner rim with pink.

3. Use **small brush** to dot sparkly fuchsia under outer corner.

4. Use **mini blender brush** to apply sparkly fuchsia to crease, blending it up.

5. Use **mini blender brush** to apply pearl to inner corners of eye, top and bottom.

6. Use **eyeliner brush** to line base of lower lashes with lapis blue.

7. Apply **mascara**.

HINT If you have round eyes, try lining the inner rim of your lower eye with blue pencil eyeliner.

We completed Julianna's makeup with deep iridescent coral lip gloss.

spring
fling

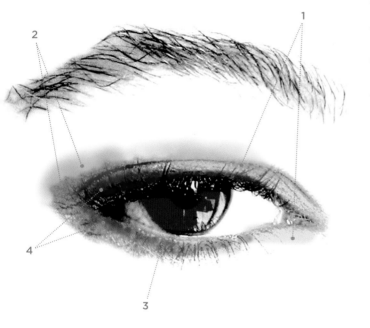

INGREDIENTS

eye shadows
iridescent pink
iridescent teal

other makeup
blue pencil eyeliner
blue cake or liquid eyeliner
black mascara

brushes
small eye shadow brush
mini blender brush
eyeliner brush

1. Use **small brush** to apply pink over inner half of upper lid to just past crease and around to inner lower corner.

2. Use **mini blender brush** to line lower lid and outer half of upper lid with teal.

3. Apply pencil **eyeliner** to inner rim of lower lash-line.

4. Use **eyeliner brush** to apply cake or liquid eyeliner very thinly along upper and lower lash-lines.

5. Apply **mascara**.

HINT If you have almond-shaped eyes, thicken the eyeliner very slightly in the outer corner.

Jonelli's look was completed with reddish-brown cream blush and soft, pearly pink lip gloss.

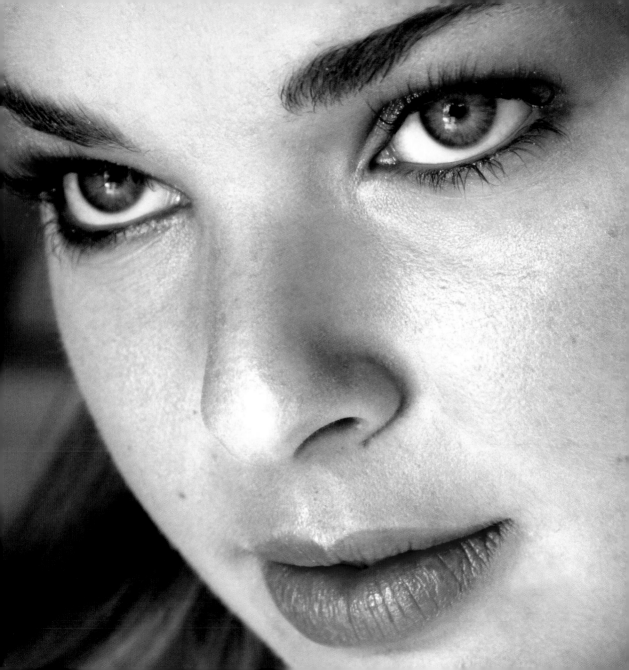

colorful

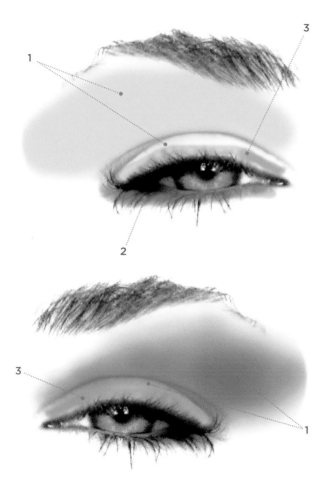

INGREDIENTS

eye shadows
iridescent orange
iridescent pink
iridescent purple
iridescent beige

other makeup
black mascara

brushes
wide eye shadow
mini blender brush

1. Use **wide brush** to blend orange over upper lid and brow bone on the right eye; pink on the left eye.

2. Use **mini blender brush** to line lower lid of right eye with purple.

3. Use **mini blender brush** to line both upper lids with beige.

4. Apply **mascara**.

HINT Another great combination would be to use green on one eye, blue on the other, and yellow underneath.

To complete Nicole's look, we added vibrant pink cream blush and berry lip gloss.

funky

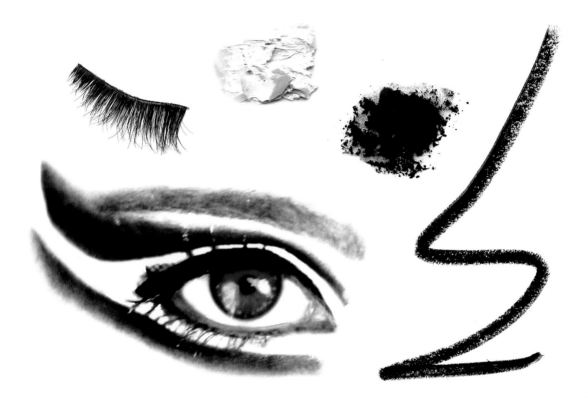

Funky can be anything that is a little over-the-top or off the beaten path. It can be soft—such as light, mascara-less lashes and pastel-colored lids— or outrageously strong, with brightly colored lids and double-layer lashes. Anything goes!

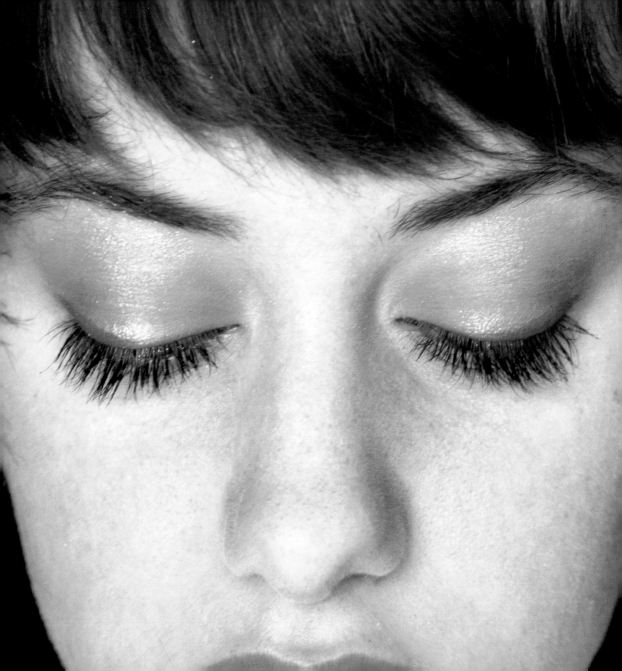

neon

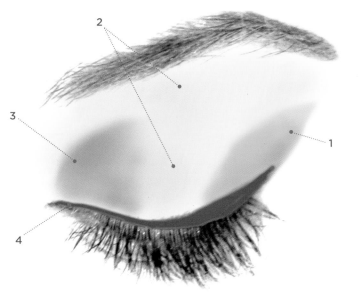

INGREDIENTS

eye shadows
iridescent orange
iridescent yellow
iridescent lime
iridescent pink

other makeup
brown or black mascara

brushes
wide eye shadow brush
large eye shadow brush
small eye shadow brush
eyeliner brush

1. Use **wide brush** to apply orange over outer upper lid and brow bone, blending out.

2. Use **large brush** to blend yellow over inner two-thirds of upper lid and brow bone, blending into orange.

3. Use **small bush** to apply lime to inner corner of eye.

4. Wet **eyeliner brush** and use it to line upper lash-line with pink.

5. Apply **mascara**.

HINT If you have dark eyes, trying switching the palette to blue, aqua, and green shadows with a violet eyeliner.

We completed Amy's look with hot pink lipstick.

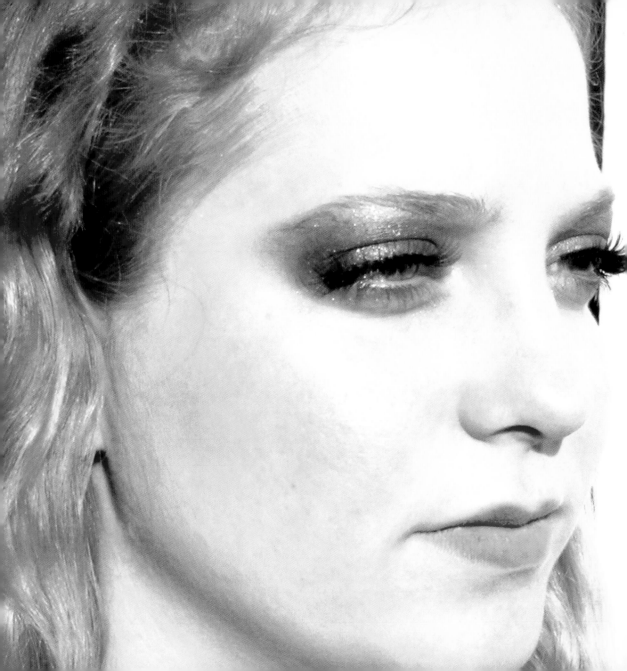

electric

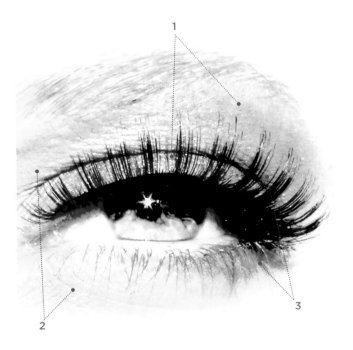

eye shadows
matte hot pink
iridescent lavender
semimatte yellow
semimatte green

other makeup
brown mascara or
    brown false eyelashes

brushes
wide eye shadow brush
small eye shadow brush
mini blender brush

1. Use **wide brush** to apply hot pink to upper lid and brow bone. Then soften by covering with a layer of lavender.

2. Use **small brush** to blend yellow under eye and in inner corner of upper lid.

3. Use **mini blender brush** to add green to outer crease and around lower eye.

4. Apply **mascara**, or **falsies** (shown here) for extra strength.

HINT If you want, apply a little lavender over the green and yellow to tone down the look.

We finished Beth's look with soft pink cream blush blended over the apples of her cheeks and hot pink lipstick (used delicately so as not to distract from the eyes).

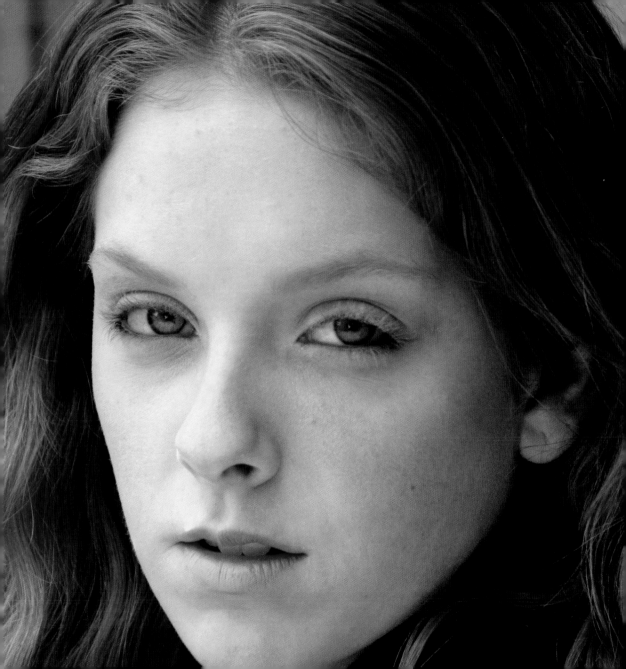

urban
poet

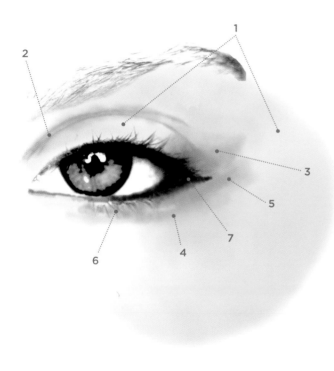

INGREDIENTS

eye shadows
iridescent light rose
matte hot pink
semimatte yellow
semimatte turquoise

other makeup
dark gray pencil eyeliner

brushes
blusher brush
mini blender brush
small eye shadow brush

1. Use **blusher brush** to apply rose all around lid and brow and onto cheekbone in one swipe.

2. Use **mini blender brush** to apply hot pink to inner crease.

3. Use **mini blender brush** to apply hot pink in outer corner of upper lid.

4. Use **mini blender brush** to apply hot pink under eye.

5. Use **small brush** to dot yellow along outer corner of lower lash-line, extending past eye.

6. Use **mini blender brush** to add turquoise under center of eye.

7. Apply **eyeliner** to inner rim of lower eye, extending it slightly past eye.

HINT Blondes and redheads may want to define their brows with a blonde brow pencil. Dark brunettes may want to lighten their lashes by powdering them with rose eye shadow to retain the ethereal feel of this look.

Suzanne's look was finished with a touch of hot pink lipstick.

moulin rouge

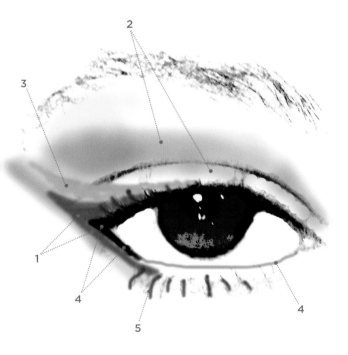

INGREDIENTS

eye shadows
matte red
iridescent green
semimatte yellow

other makeup
black pencil eyeliner
blue mascara

brushes
eyeliner brush
small eye shadow brush
mini blender brush

1. Use **eyeliner brush** to apply red to outer corners, following the line of eye.

2. Use **small brush** to apply green to upper lid, going just past crease and blending out to brow, following line of red shadow.

3. Use **mini blender brush** to draw yellow line above red, blending it lightly into green.

4. Line inner rim of lower eye with **eyeliner**. Also line outer parts of upper and lower lids.

5. Apply **mascara**.

HINT Keep the eye elegant by applying the red shadow very delicately and to just the outer corner of the eye. Also, if you have pale skin and want to make this look subtler, try brown eyeliner instead of the red shadow.

We completed Jonelli's look with reddish-brown cream blush and a touch of iridescent pink lip gloss.

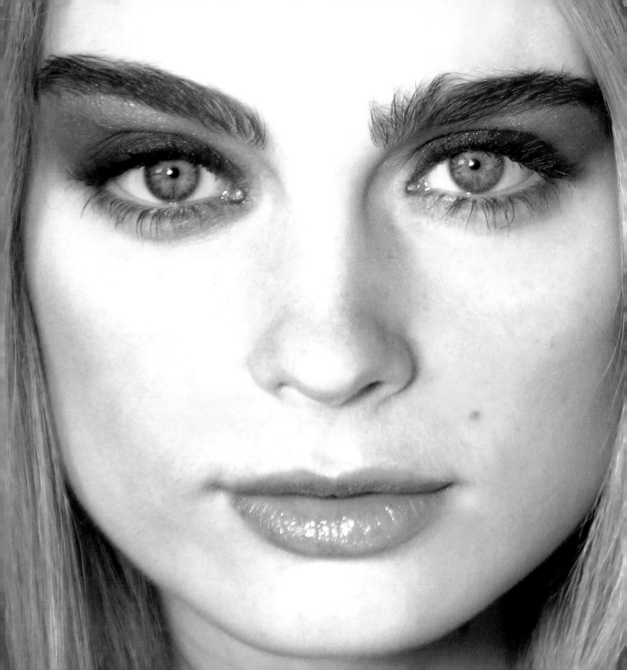

firestarter

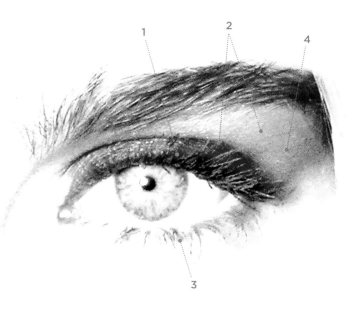

INGREDIENTS

eye shadows
iridescent red
iridescent dusty pink

other makeup
red pencil eyeliner
black and green mascara

brushes
wide eye shadow brush
eyeliner brush
small eye shadow brush

1. Line upper lid with **eyeliner**.

2. Use **wide brush** to apply red shadow over upper lid and brow bone, covering the eyeliner.

3. Use **eyeliner brush** to apply touch of red shadow along lower lash-line.

4. Use **small brush** to dot dusty pink on brow bone for a highlight.

5. Apply **black mascara** to one eye and **green mascara** to the other—this is a very subtle way of attracting attention.

HINT Try this mascara trick with soft neutral makeup and see who notices!

To complete Laurenne's makeup, we used a touch of coral blush and clear lip gloss.

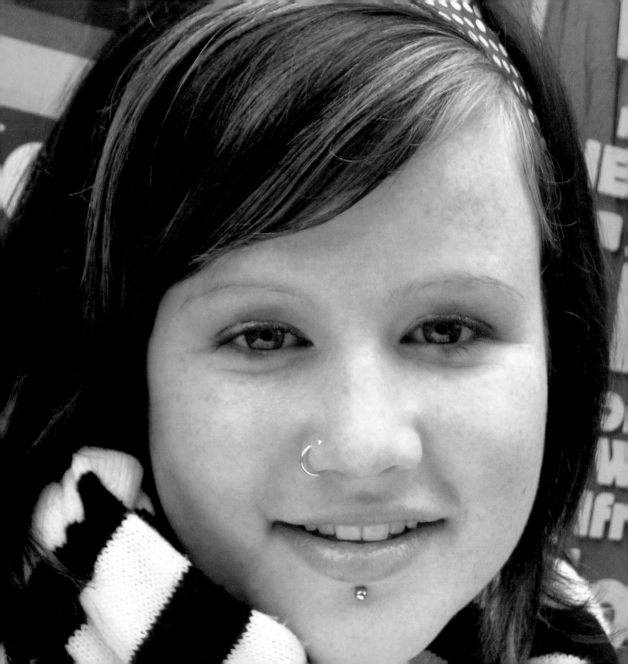

playful

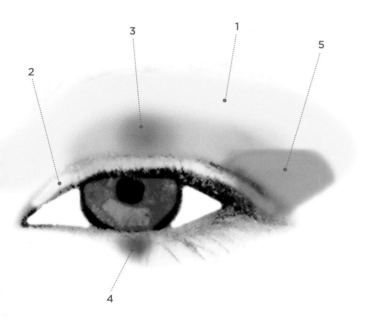

eye shadows
iridescent pink
metallic silver
matte violet
matte lapis blue

other makeup
black mascara

brushes
wide eye shadow brush
mini blender brush

1. Use **wide brush** to apply pink to brow bone.

2. Use **mini blender brush** to apply silver over inner two-thirds of upper lid.

3. Use **mini blender brush** to apply large dot of violet above crease.

4. Use **mini blender brush** to add small dot of violet below center of eye.

5. Use **mini blender brush** to apply lapis blue to outer corner of upper lid, from lash-line to just above crease.

6. Apply **mascara**.

HINT If you want something more conservative, change the violet dot under the eye to blue. For something more daring, place three dots of color under the eye. You can also try this look with orange, red, and gold shadows instead.

We finished Lisa's makeup with a touch of coral blush and iridescent pink lip gloss.

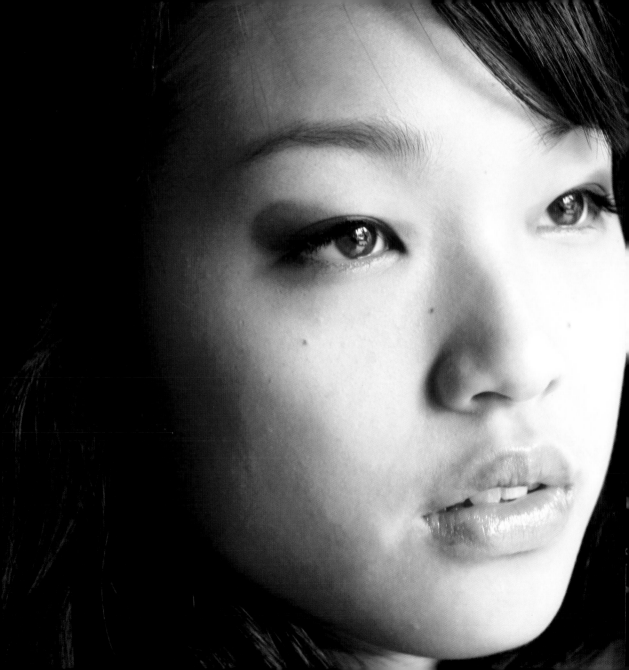

beatnik

INGREDIENTS

eye shadows
matte orange
matte deep green

other makeup
black mascara

brushes
small eye shadow brush
mini blender brush

1. Use **mini blender brush** to apply touch of orange to inner corner of eye.

2. Use **small brush** to press deep green into outer corner. Don't blend the colors!

3. Apply **mascara**.

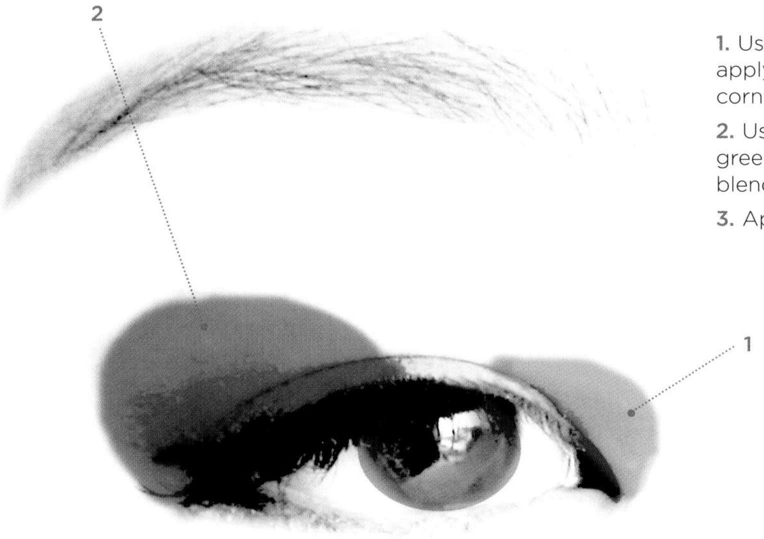

2

1

HINT To pump up this look, add bright orange lip color.

We finished Ming's look with yellow lip gloss and white pearl lipstick.

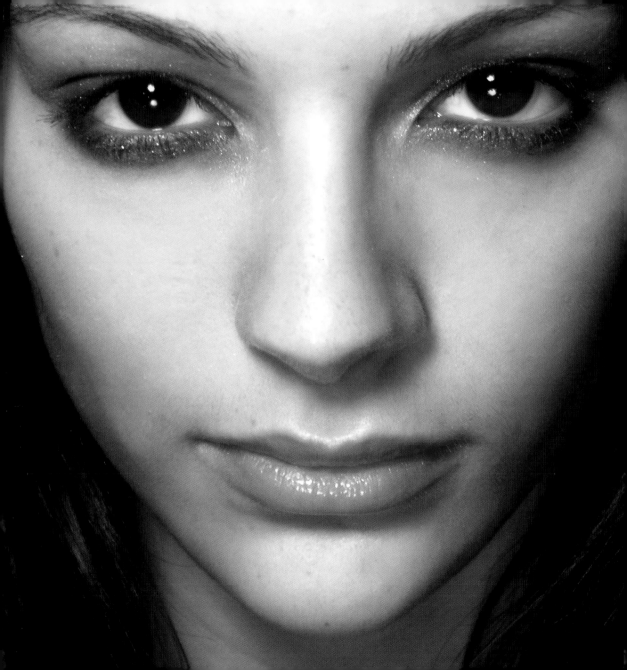

bejeweled

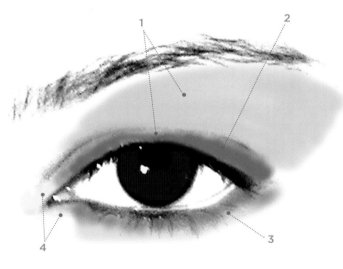

eye shadows
semimatte acid green
iridescent bright green
iridescent purple
iridescent pale green

other makeup
black mascara

brushes
large eye shadow brush
mini blender brush
eyeliner brush

1. Use **large brush** to blend acid green over upper lid and brow bone.

2. Use **mini blender brush** to apply bright green on upper lid to just past crease, blending up and out.

3. Use **mini blender brush** to line lower lid with purple.

4. Use **eyeliner brush** to add touch of pale green to inner corners.

5. Finish with **mascara**.

HINT To strengthen this look, use violet pencil eyeliner to line the inner rim of the lower eye.

We completed Marisol's look with reddish-brown cream blush and coral lipstick topped with clear gloss.

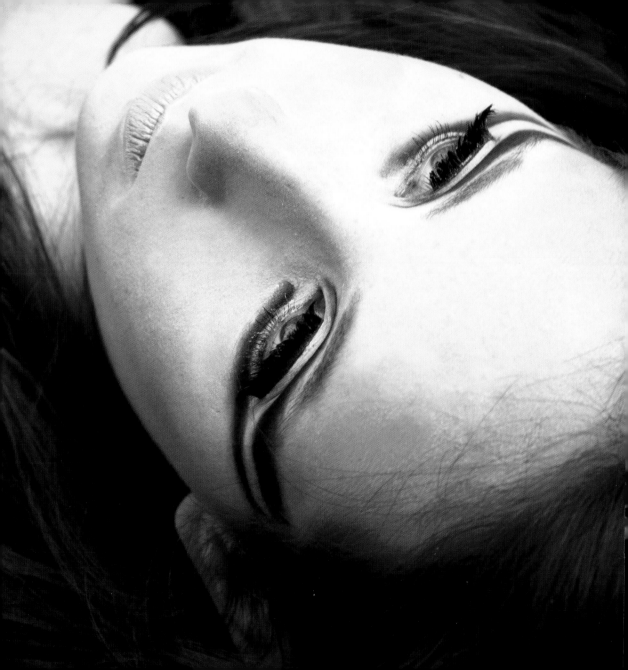

odyssey

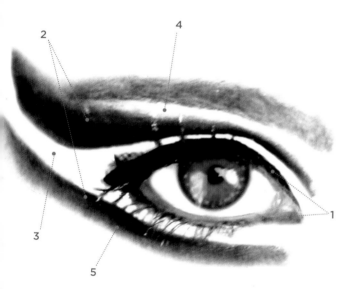

INGREDIENTS

eye shadows
cream white
matte black

other makeup
black pencil eyeliner
translucent powder
black mascara, or black
    false eyelashes

brushes
mini blender brush
synthetic concealer brush
wide eye shadow brush
small eye shadow brush

1. Line upper and lower lids with **eyeliner.**

2. Draw zebra stripes with eyeliner, as shown, and then smudge lines with **mini blender brush.**

3. Apply white with **synthetic brush**, filling in area around eye between black zebra stripes.

4. Use **synthetic brush** to add more white under brow.

5. Use **wide brush** to lightly dust **translucent powder** over eye to set.

6. Use **small eye shadow brush** to blend black shadow over black zebra lines.

7. Apply **mascara**, or falsies.

HINT This eye is very dramatic on pale skin. You can lighten your skin by blending a white base with your usual base. Those with darker complexions might try this look with bronze and silver instead.

We gave Rachel's lips a retro 1960s feel with a light pink lip color made by mixing white eye shadow and pink lipstick. A touch of red under the cheekbones completed the look.

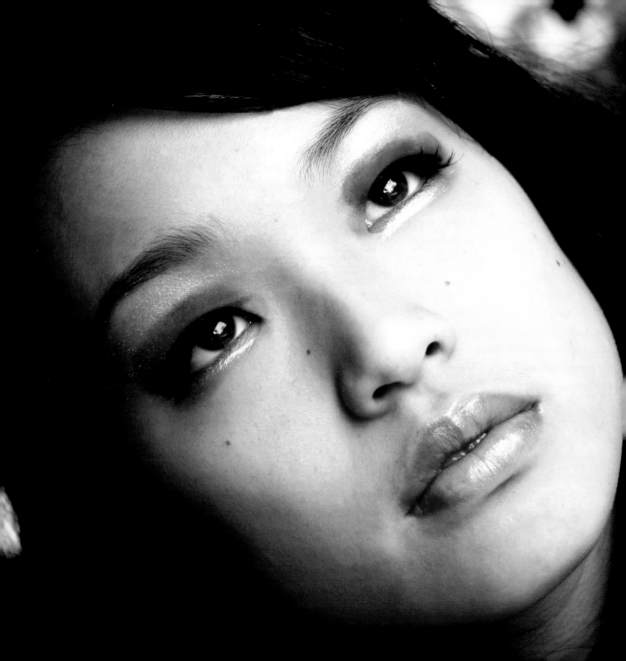

abstraction

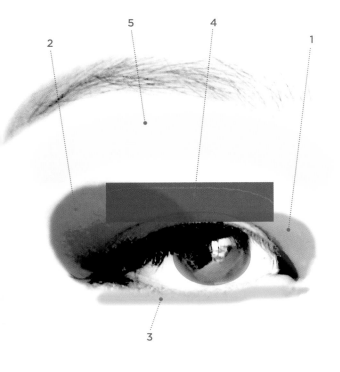

eye shadows
matte orange
matte deep green
metallic silver
iridescent yellow

other makeup
blue cake eyeliner
black mascara

brushes
mini blender brush
small eye shadow brush
synthetic concealer brush
large eye shadow brush

1. Use **mini blender brush** to apply a touch of orange to inner corner of eye.

2. Use **small brush** to press deep green into outer corner.

3. Use **mini blender brush** to add stripe of silver under eye (wipe off any orange from your brush first).

4. Dip **synthetic brush** in water and then use its flat edge to sweep eyeliner across lid.

5. Use **large brush** to add a delicate touch of yellow under brow.

6. Apply **mascara**.

HINT Apply the silver eye shadow under your eyes with a wet brush if you want to make it stronger.

We finished Ming's look with yellow lip gloss.

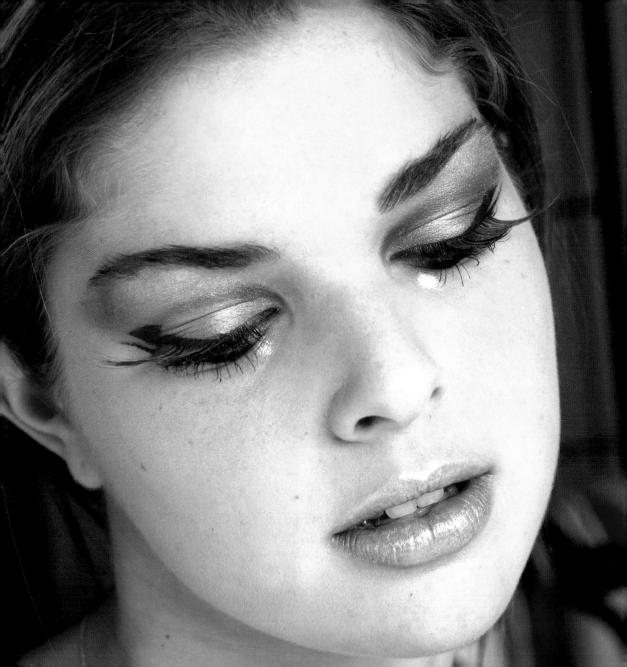

vanity

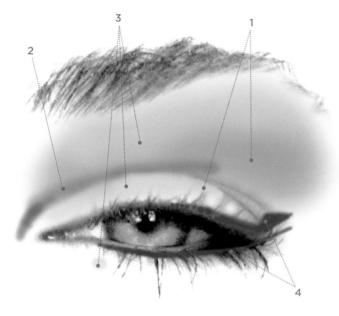

INGREDIENTS

eye shadows
iridescent medium aqua
iridescent lapis blue
iridescent pale aqua

other makeup
blue cake or liquid eyeliner
blue false eyelashes (or black
   ones and blue mascara)

brushes
wide eye shadow brush
mini blender brush
small eye shadow brush
eyeliner brush

1. Use **wide brush** to blend medium aqua over upper lid and brow bone.

2. Use **mini blender blush** to line crease with lapis blue, starting darker in the inner corner and getting lighter as you go.

3. Use **small brush** to add a touch of pale aqua to center of lid and brow bone. Also add a dot under eye.

4. Use **eyeliner brush** to line lower lid and outer half of upper lid with eyeliner, winging up as shown.

5. Apply **blue falsies**. If you don't have blue falsies, use **black** ones and apply lots of **blue mascara** to them.

HINT If you can't find this eyelash shape, cut a pair of regular lashes in half and apply only the inner halves to the outer part of your eyes.

Nicole's look was completed with rose blush and soft pearly pink lip gloss.

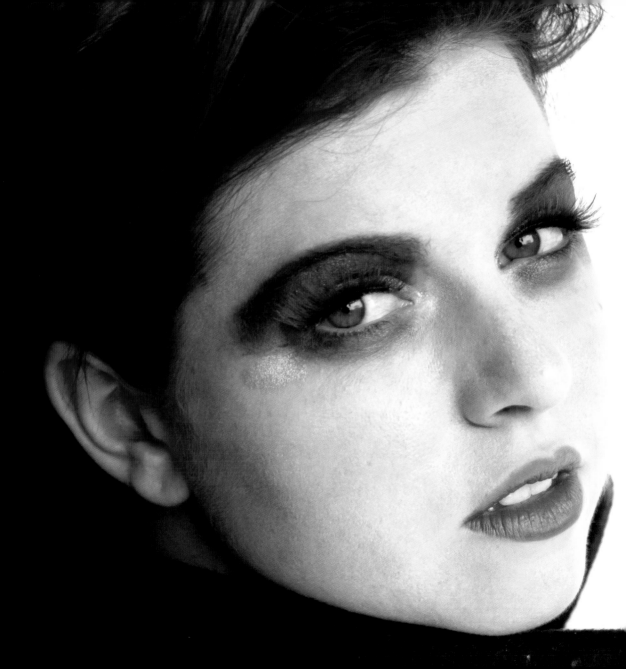

mardi gras

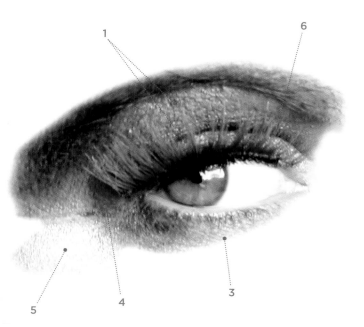

INGREDIENTS

eye shadows
cream iridescent pale green
iridescent olive
iridescent navy blue
iridescent lavender
iridescent aqua

other makeup
blue cake eyeliner
green and yellow false eyelashes

brushes
synthetic concealer brush
small eye shadow brush
mini blender brush

1. Use your **fingertips** or **synthetic brush** to blend a very thin layer of pale green over upper lid and brow bone.

2. Press various powder shadows into cream with the **small** and **mini blender brushes.** You can follow diagram or make up your own.

3. Blend lavender with **mini blender brush** under eye.

4. Wet **synthetic brush** and dab outer corner of eye with **eyeliner.**

5. Smudge pale green in outer corner with **mini blender brush.**

6. Apply **green falsies** to very base of upper lashes. Then apply **yellow falsies** on top of them.

HINT Whiten your face first to make the eye colors pop even more. Also, if you have blue eyes, try blue and yellow falsies; if you have dark eyes, try red and yellow falsies.

We completed Kristen's look with red matte lipstick.

glamorous

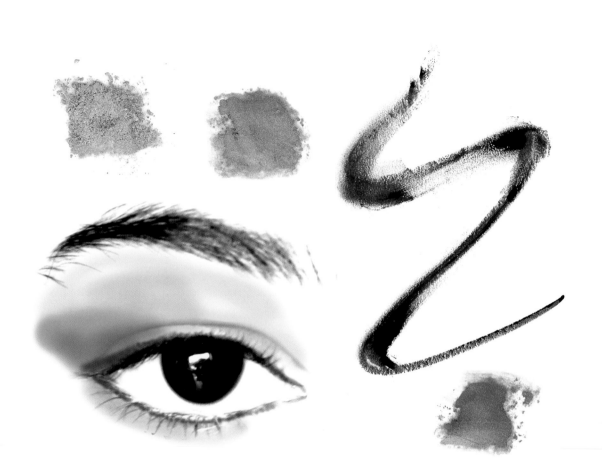

Glamorous is deep and mysterious, sometimes monochromatic, and always stunning. It can range from dark matte colors to shimmering pearls—but no timid in-betweens. No matter which way you go, you will not be forgotten!

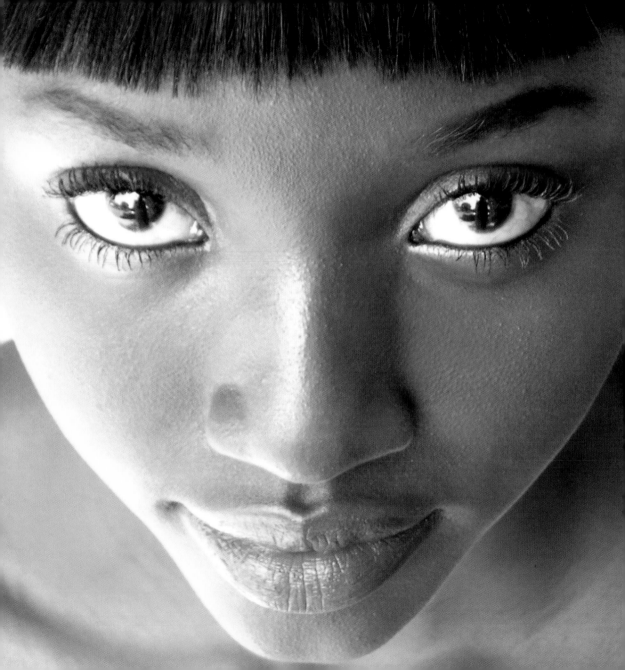

bright
eyes

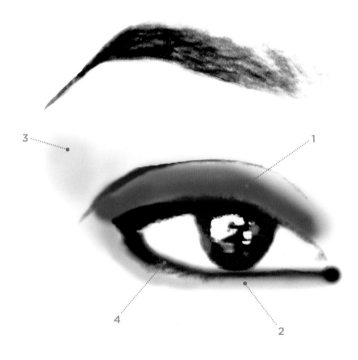

INGREDIENTS

eye shadows
iridescent lapis blue
iridescent pale green

other makeup
black pencil eyeliner
black mascara

brushes
mini blender brush
eyeliner brush

1. Use **mini blender brush** to apply lapis blue on upper lid, from lash-line to crease.

2. Use **eyeliner brush** to line lower lid with pale green.

3. Use **mini blender brush** to blend a touch of pale green on outer brow bone just above lapis blue.

4. Line inner rim of lower eye with **eyeliner**.

5. Apply **mascara**.

HINT If your eyes are not a perfect almond shape, put a touch of black eyeliner along the outer corner of your upper lash-line to give them an extra lift.

To finish Rose's regal look, we used bright pink cream blush and vibrant pink lipstick.

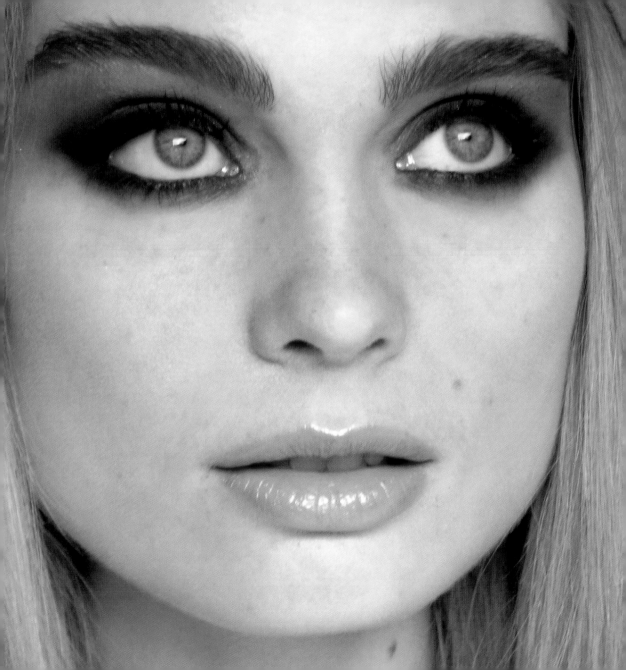

oomph

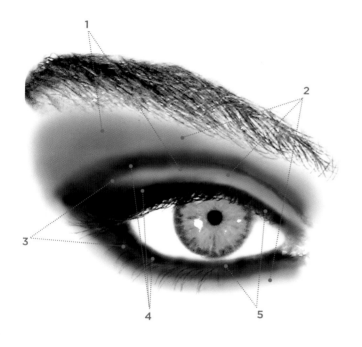

INGREDIENTS

eye shadows
semimatte taupe
matte yellow-brown
matte gray
matte dark brown
matte black

other makeup
black pencil eyeliner
black mascara

brushes
wide eye shadow brush
small eye shadow brush
mini blender brush
eyeliner brush

1. Use **wide brush** to dust taupe over upper lid and brow bone.

2. Use **wide brush** to layer yellow-brown over upper lid and brow bone, as well as under eye.

3. Use **small brush** to apply gray on upper lid, just up to the crease, and under eye.

4. Use **mini blender brush** to apply dark brown along upper and lower lash-lines over the other colors, in a slightly narrower line. Also apply to crease.

5. Line inner rim of lower eye and upper lash-line with **eyeliner**.

6. Use **eyeliner brush** to blend black shadow over eyeliner along upper lash-line.

7. Finish with lots of **mascara**.

HINT When you blend, keep the shadows strongest at the outer part of the lid; don't go too heavy in the inner corners. To soften the look, finish by blending a final layer of taupe over the entire lid.

We kept the attention on Laurenne's eyes by finishing with taupe blush and nude lipstick topped with yellow gloss.

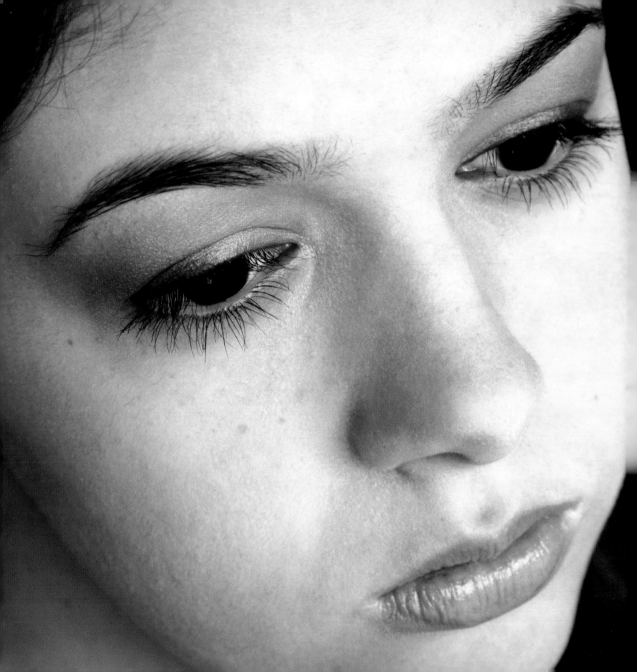

blue
mood

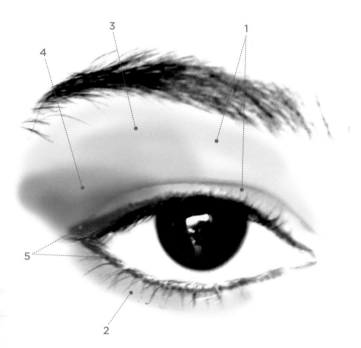

INGREDIENTS

eye shadows
iridescent pale aqua
iridescent medium aqua
semimatte turquoise

other makeup
blue-green pencil eyeliner
black mascara

brushes
large eye shadow brush
small eye shadow brush

1. Use **large brush** to apply pale aqua over upper lid and brow bone.

2. Use **large brush** to apply pale aqua under eye.

3. Use **small brush** to apply medium aqua above upper lid.

4. Use **small brush** to blend turquoise from outer corner to center of upper lid, making a smooth transition.

5. Line lower lid and outer part of upper lid delicately with **eyeliner**.

6. Apply **mascara**.

HINT To strengthen this eye, blend a matte deep green shadow into the outer corner of the lid.

We completed Lexi's look with a touch of coral blush high on the cheeks and soft pink lip color.

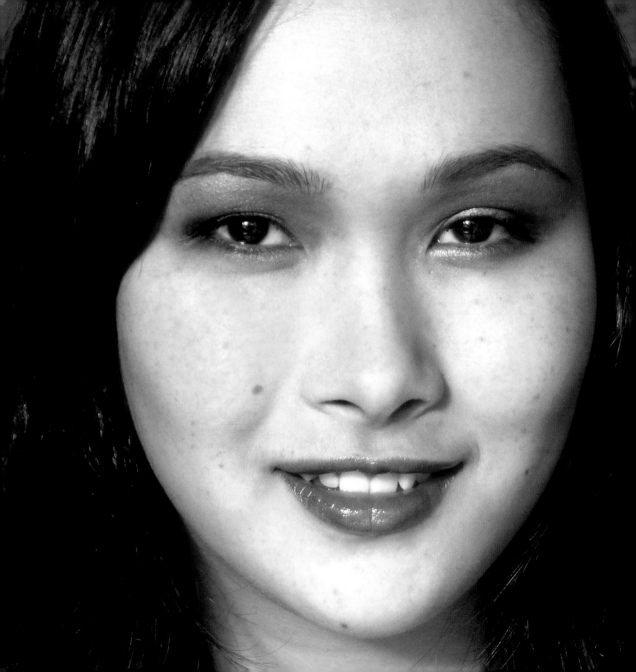

exotic

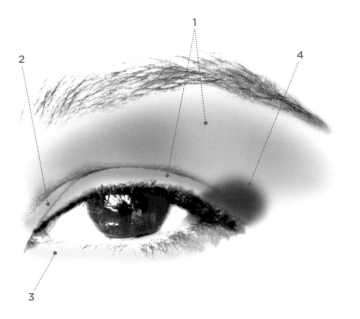

INGREDIENTS

eye shadows
cream tarnished gold
iridescent pale gold
matte lapis blue

other makeup
black mascara

brushes
small eye shadow brush
mini blender brush (optional)

1. Use your **fingertip** to blend tarnished gold over upper lid and brow bone.

2. Use **small brush** to add pale gold to inner corner of upper lid.

3. Use **small brush** to line lower eye with pale gold.

4. Use your **fingertip** or **mini blender brush** to dot lapis blue in outer corner of upper lid.

5. Apply **mascara**.

HINT To help this look last longer, finish by dusting your lids with a layer of translucent powder.

To finish Paula's look, we added bright pink cream blush on the apples of her cheeks and berry lip gloss.

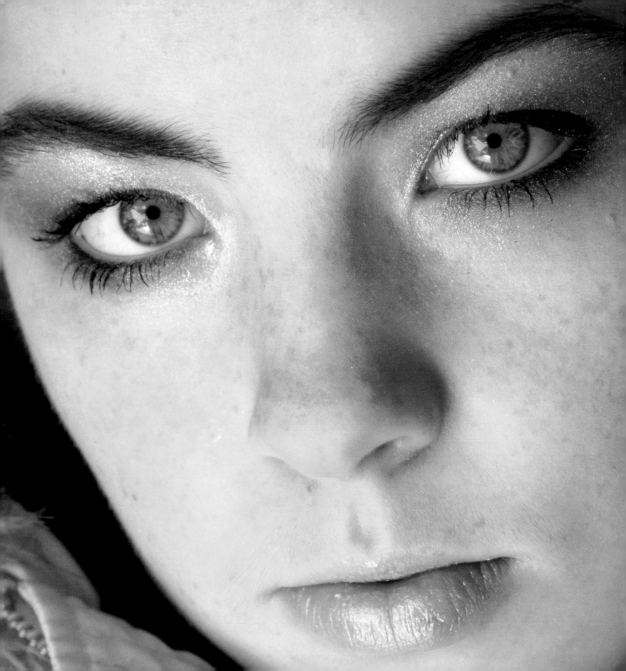

celestial

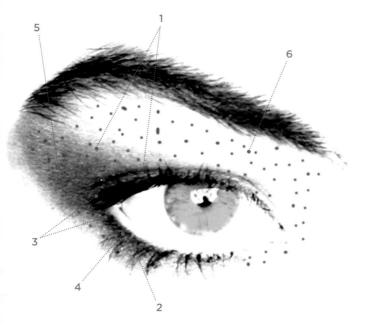

INGREDIENTS

eye shadows
iridescent navy
matte black
iridescent pearl

other makeup
black pencil eyeliner
black mascara

brushes
wide eye shadow brush
small eye shadow brush
large eye shadow brush

1. Use **wide brush** to apply navy to upper lid, going past the crease and blending it up and out to brow.

2. Use **wide brush** to apply navy along lower lid.

3. Use **small brush** to blend black over the navy at base of upper and lower lashes. Then blend out.

4. Delicately line lower lid with **eyeliner**.

5. Use **small brush** to blend more black shadow into outer part of eye, on top and bottom and from base of lashes outward.

6. Use **large brush** to dust pearl over entire upper and lower lid areas (area covered with red dots).

7. Apply **mascara**.

HINT Use a deep burgundy lip color to make this look even more dramatic.

We finished Alana's look with soft pink cream blush and iridescent pink lip gloss.

knockout

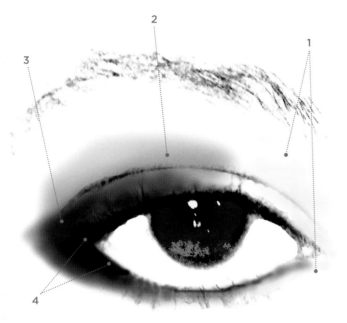

INGREDIENTS

eye shadows
iridescent pale lilac
matte dark gray
matte black

other makeup
black pencil eyeliner
black mascara

brushes
small eye shadow brush
wide eye shadow brush

1. Use **small brush** to apply pale lilac to inner half of upper lid and along inner part of lower lid.

2. Use **wide brush** to apply dark gray to outer half of upper lid, overlapping the pale lilac a little.

3. Use **small brush** to blend black into outer top and bottom corners, blending it into and over the gray.

4. Line upper and lower lids with **eyeliner**.

5. Apply **mascara**.

HINT You need great brows with this eye, so don't forget to define them!

We finished Jonelli's look with reddish-brown blush and nude lipstick.

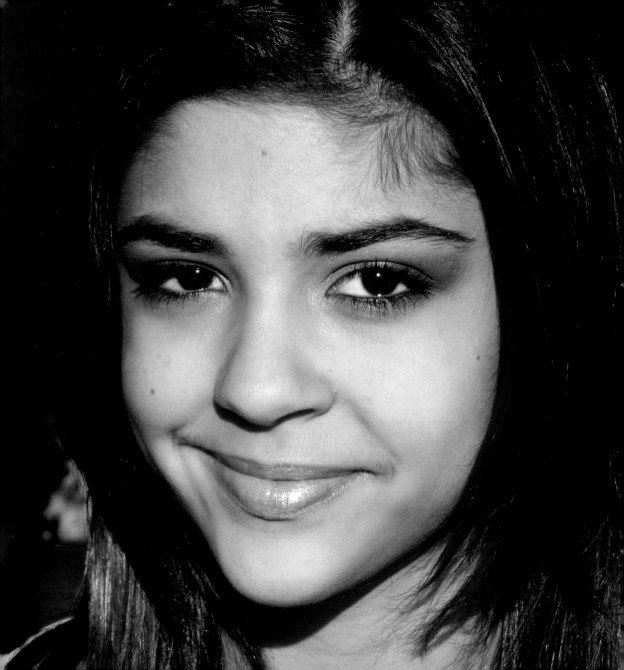

zingara

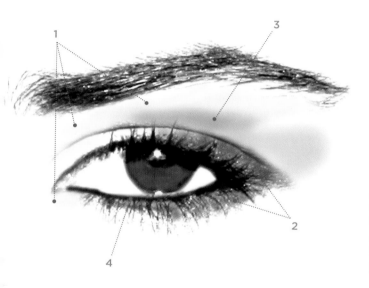

INGREDIENTS

eye shadows
iridescent pale green
matte sparkly dark green
semimatte turquoise

other makeup
black pencil eyeliner
black mascara

brushes
large eye shadow brush
small eye shadow brush
mini blender brush

1. Use **large brush** to blend pale green over upper lid, brow bone, and under eye.

2. Use **small brush** to apply sparkly dark green along outer half of upper and lower lash-lines, blending it up and out.

3. Use **mini blender brush** to apply turquoise to center of upper lid, softening transition from pale to darker shades.

4. Line inner rim of lower eye with **eyeliner**.

5. Apply **mascara**.

HINT For more contrast, use bright blue eyeliner instead of black.

Savvy's look was completed with reddish-brown cream blush and soft pearly pink lip gloss.

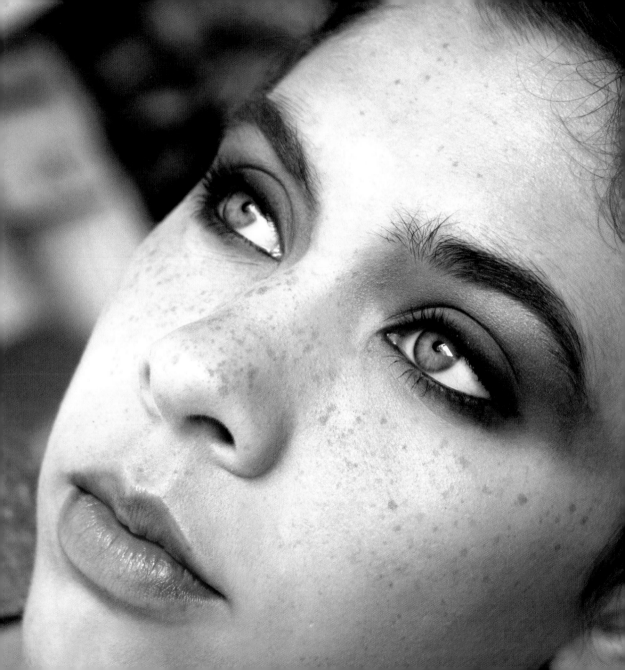

royal

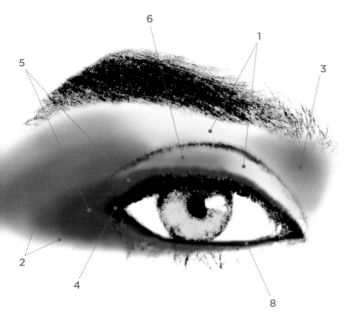

INGREDIENTS

eye shadows
cream medium lilac
matte violet
matte dark purple
iridescent pale lilac

other makeup
black pencil eyeliner
black mascara

brushes
synthetic concealer brush
small eye shadow brush
eyeliner brush
mini blender brush
large eye shadow brush

1. Use **synthetic brush** to blend medium lilac over upper lid and brow bone.

2. Use **small brush** to blend violet into outer parts of upper and lower lids.

3. Use **small brush** to apply touch of violet to inner corner of eye.

4. Use **eyeliner brush** to line upper lid with eyeliner.

5. Use **mini blender brush** to blend dark purple along upper and lower lash-lines outward and upward into violet.

6. Use **small brush** to add pale lilac highlight to center of lid.

7. Blend all colors gently with **large brush**.

8. Line inner rim of lower eye with eyeliner.

9. Apply **mascara**.

HINT If you have round eyes, elongate them by making the lilac highlight in step 6 very, very narrow.

We completed Daisy's look with berry blush and pink lipstick.

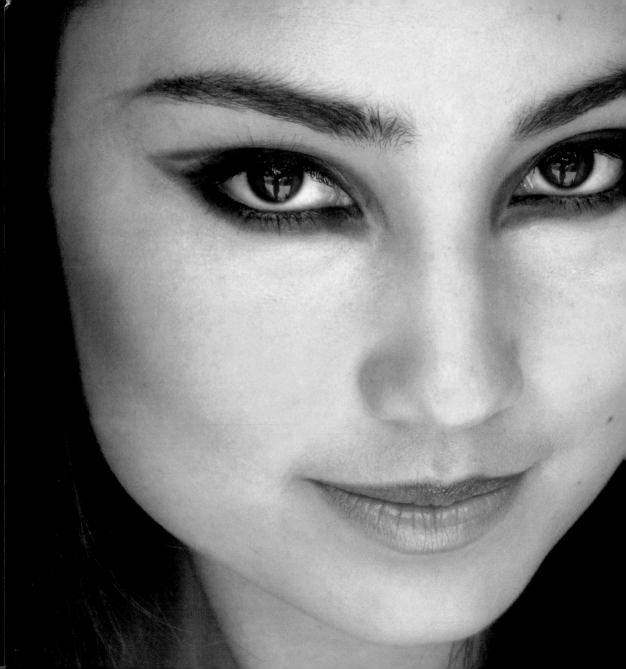

warrior

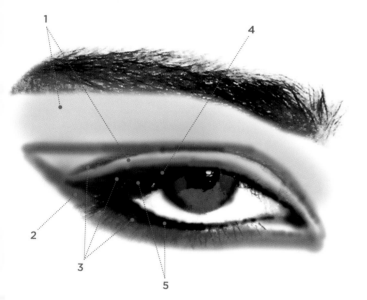

INGREDIENTS

eye shadows
semimatte yellow
matte reddish-brown
matte khaki
matte black

other makeup
black pencil eyeliner
black mascara
black individual or cluster false
  eyelashes (optional)

brushes
wide eye shadow brush
small eye shadow brush
mini blender brush
eyeliner brush

1. Use **wide brush** to cover upper lid and brow bone with yellow.

2. Use **small brush** to blend reddish-brown all around eye, creating shape as shown. Make it stronger in both inner and outer corners.

3. Use **mini blender brush** to line lower lid and outer half of upper lid with khaki. Also line crease with khaki, extending line to join reddish-brown.

4. Use **eyeliner brush** to dab black shadow along upper lash-line in very base of lashes.

5. Use **eyeliner** to line inner rim of lower eye and along upper lash-line.

6. Apply **mascara** and a few individual or cluster falsies (if desired) to upper lashes.

HINT Blend a light layer of iridescent rosy gold over the entire eyelid to soften the lines.

We lined Katrina's lips with brown pencil and dabbed a touch of red lipstick in the center.

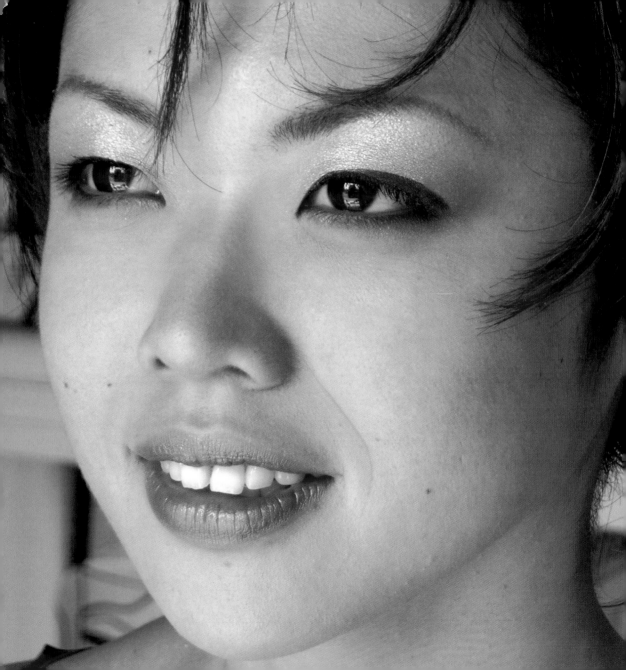

x factor

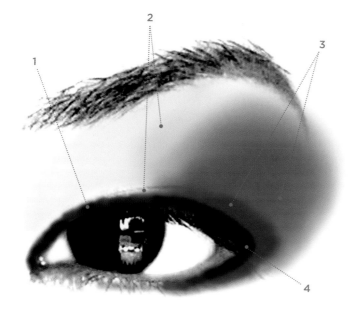

INGREDIENTS

eye shadows
iridescent pale green
iridescent olive
matte black

other makeup
black pencil eyeliner
black mascara

brushes
large eye shadow brush
wide eye shadow brush
mini blender brush

1. Line upper and lower lids with **eyeliner**.

2. Use **large brush** to apply pale green over upper lid and brow bone.

3. Use **wide brush** to apply and blend olive on outer parts of upper and lower lids.

4. Use **mini blender brush** to dab black shadow over eyeliner in outer corner of eye.

5. Finish with **mascara**.

HINT Add a touch of brown eye shadow over the black eyeliner and under the eye to soften this look.

To finish Akiko's look we added a touch of orange lip gloss.

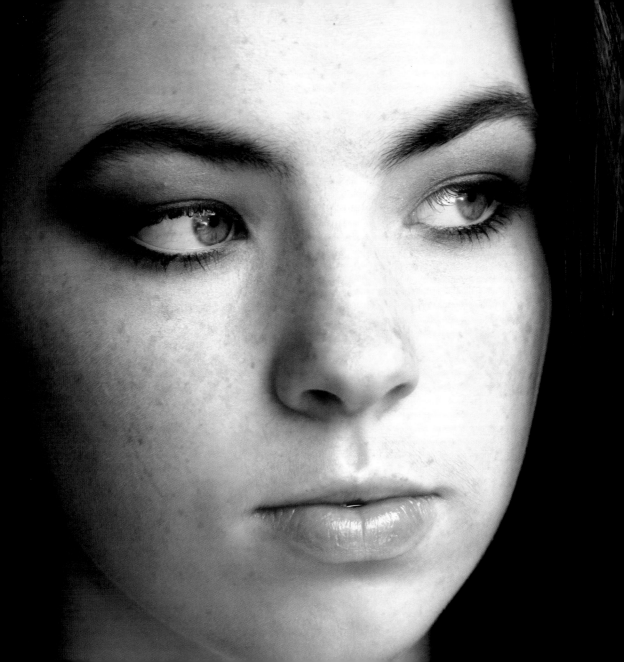

midnight

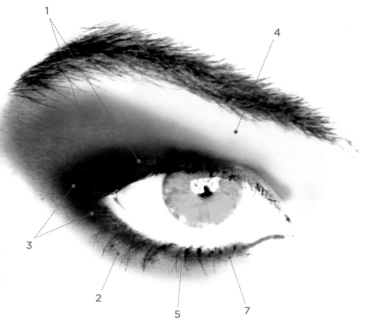

eye shadows
iridescent navy
matte black
semimatte light blue

other makeup
black pencil eyeliner
black mascara
white pencil eyeliner

brushes
wide eye shadow brush
small eye shadow brush
large eye shadow brush

1. Use **wide brush** to apply navy to upper lid, going past crease and blending up and out to brow.

2. Use **wide brush** to apply navy along lower lid.

3. Use **small brush** to blend black over the navy in base of upper and lower lashes, blending out.

4. Use **large brush** to blend light blue on brow bone. Add a touch under eye as well.

5. Delicately line lower lid with **black pencil eyeliner**.

6. Apply **mascara**.

7. Line inner rim of lower lash-line with **white pencil eyeliner**.

HINT Apply blue pencil eyeliner to the inner rim of the lower eye to intensify this look.

We finished Alana's look with soft pink cream blush and iridescent pink lip gloss.

inspired

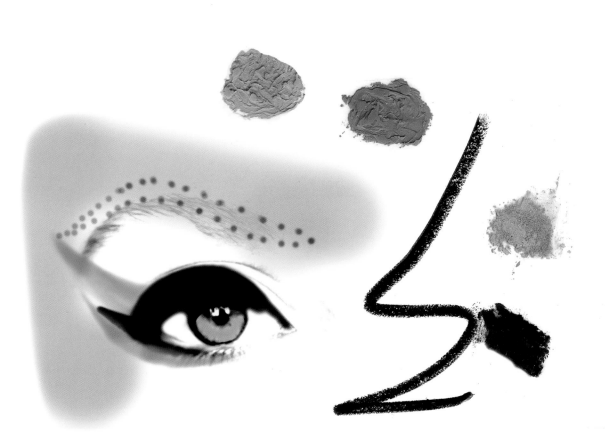

Makeup artists are constantly being inspired by the world around us. The face of a glamorous movie star, a painting in a museum, the colors of a wildflower garden—these things and more drive our creative spirits and find a way into our looks. Here are ten of my personal inspirations, with a tribute to each. What inspires *you*?

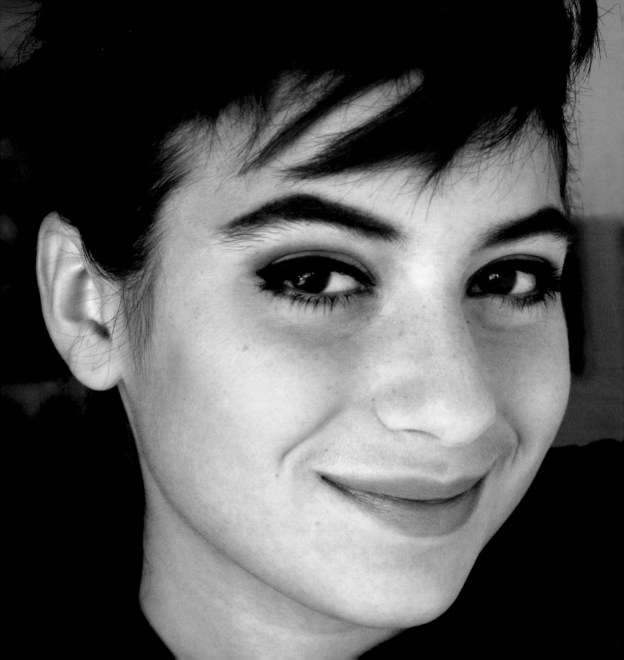

audrey hepburn

Born May 4, 1929, in Belgium, Audrey Hepburn became a star of the stage and screen in the 1950s and 60s, as well a legendary symbol of glamour and style. Having trained as a ballerina before pursuing acting, she had exceptional grace as well as a fresh, youthful elegance. From 1988 until her death in 1993, Audrey served as a UNICEF goodwill ambassador and received the Presidential Medal of Freedom for her work. This look is inspired by her trademark eyeliner, brows, and pixie elegance.

INGREDIENTS

eye shadows
matte khaki
matte white

other makeup
brown brow pencil
black cake eyeliner
black mascara

brushes
mini blender brush
small eye shadow brush
angled brow brush

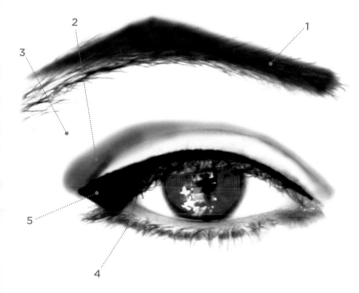

1. Thicken eyebrows with **brow pencil**. Accentuate the arch, making it slightly pointed.

2. Use **mini blender brush** to apply khaki to crease.

3. Use **small brush** to blend white on brow bone.

4. Dot **brow pencil** a little along lower lash-line.

5. Wet **angled brow brush** and load with eyeliner. Place brush flat against outer corner of eye, with longest part pointing up, and blend eyeliner to inner corner of eye.

6. Apply **mascara**.

HINT Line your upper lid with brown brow pencil first. Rub off places where you made it too thick, such as over the center of the eye and in the inner corner, with a cotton swab. Then go over the line with the angled brush and cake eyeliner.

To finish this ode to Audrey, we gave Luna a touch of coral blush and pinky beige lip color.

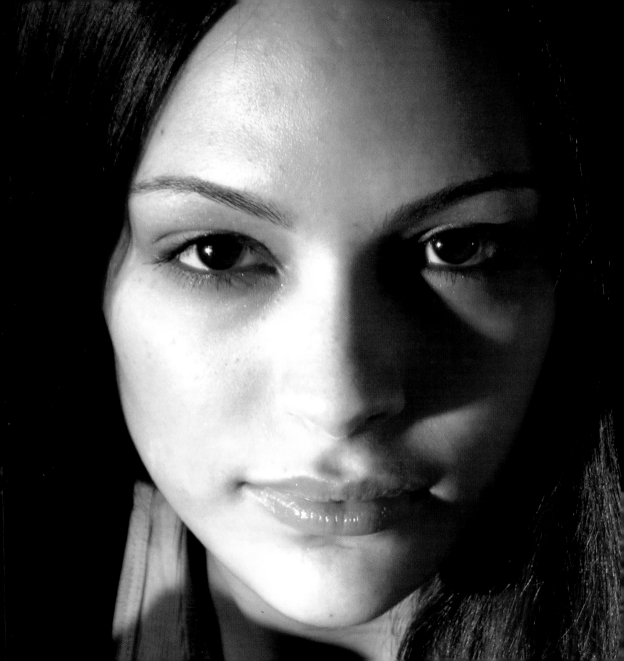

mata hari

To me, Mata Hari is a symbol of mystery and exoticism. She was born Margaretha Geertruida Zelle, in Holland, on August 7, 1876. Taking the stage name Mata Hari, she became a sensation in Paris, where she performed as an Indonesian princess practicing the art of Indian dance. During World War I, Mata Hari developed relationships with several high-ranking miliary officials and traveled frequently between warring countries. In 1917, she was arrested as a spy, and, even though there was no concrete evidence against her, was found guilty. She was executed later that year. Here we evoke the exoticism of Mata Hari's legend with a blend of monochromatic greens.

INGREDIENTS

eye shadows
semimatte acid green
iridescent green
iridescent gold-green

other makeup
black mascara

brushes
large eye shadow brush
small eye shadow brush

1. Use **large brush** to apply acid green over upper lid, brow bone, and below eye.

2. Use **small brush** to apply green from upper lid to crease, and then around to line lower lid.

3. Use **small brush** to add a gold-green highlight under brow.

4. Apply **mascara**.

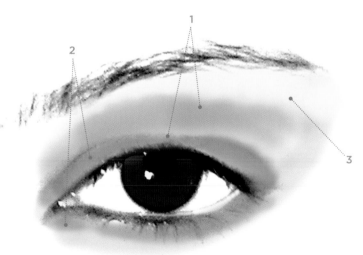

HINT If you're blonde, add more drama by lining the inner rim of your lower eye with green pencil eyeliner.

To complete our Mata Hari look, we gave Marisol soft pink cream blush and iridescent pink lip gloss.

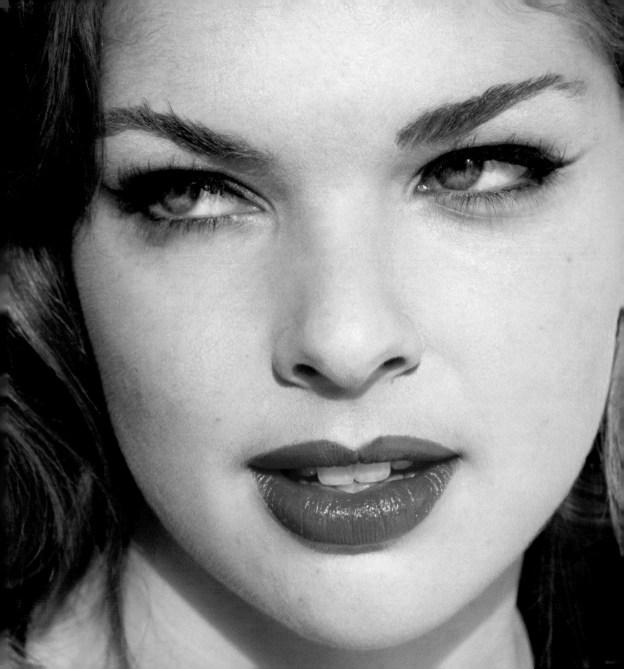

marilyn monroe

I'm hardly the only one captivated by Marilyn—her look has inspired everyone from Madonna to Anna Nicole Smith to Andy Warhol. Born June 1, 1926, as Norma Jean Mortenson, Marilyn Monroe became one of the most popular actresses of the 1950s. Famous for her beauty as well as her comedic talent and screen presence, Marilyn immortalized red lipstick and black eyeliner as symbols of classic elegance and sophistication. Here we offer our own version of her fabulous look.

INGREDIENTS

eye shadows
matte white
semimatte taupe

other makeup
black cake or liquid eyeliner
black mascara

brushes
wide eye shadow brush
mini blender brush
eyeliner brush

1. Use **wide brush** to apply white over upper lid and brow bone.

2. Use **mini blender brush** to accentuate crease with taupe.

3. Use **eyeliner brush** to apply eyeliner along upper lash-line, flicking it out and up at the end. Put a little eyeliner along outer lower lid as well, joining the upper line.

4. Finish with lots of **mascara**.

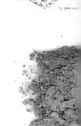

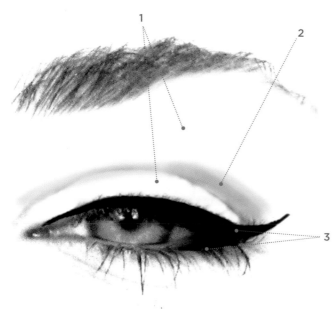

HINT To update this look, try using a colored eye shadow on the lid instead of white.

We finished this look on Nicole with a hint of red on the cheeks and a fabulous red matte lipstick.

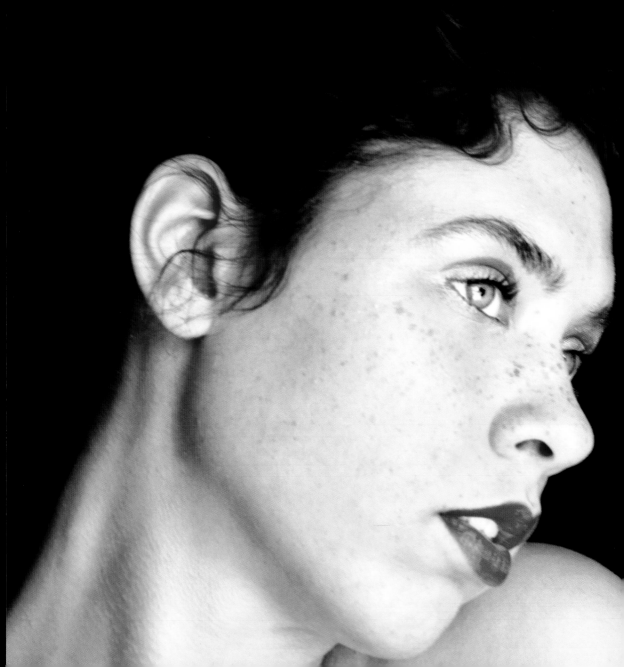

sunset

What could be more inspiring than the colors and designs found in nature? Silver stars, ever-changing oceans, and, here, a mesmerizing sunset. Look around and be inspired!

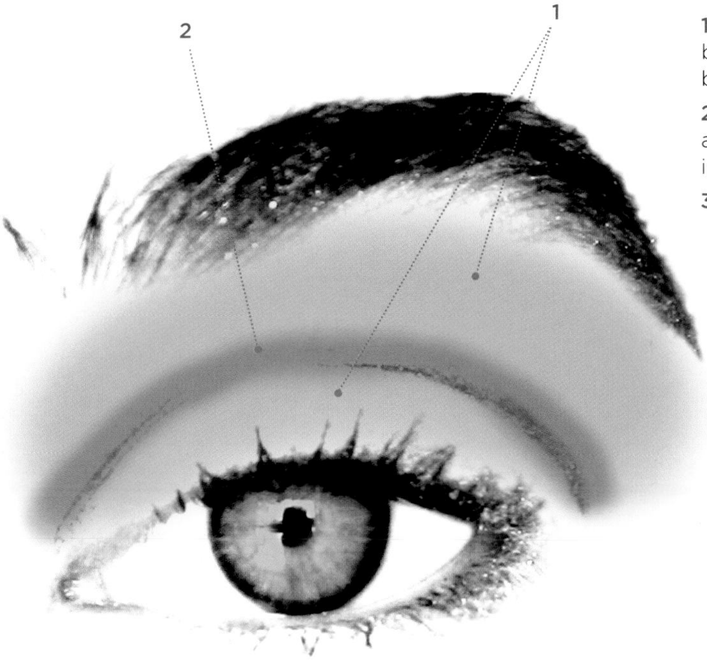

INGREDIENTS

eye shadows
iridescent bronze
matte sparkly fuchsia

other makeup
black mascara

brushes
large eye shadow brush
mini blender brush

1. Use **large brush** to dust bronze over upper lid and brow bone.

2. Wet **mini blender brush** to apply a sparkly fuchsia line in crease.

3. Apply **mascara**.

2

1

HINT   Color the brows orange for more intensity.

We completed Daisy's look with a strong deep red lip color.

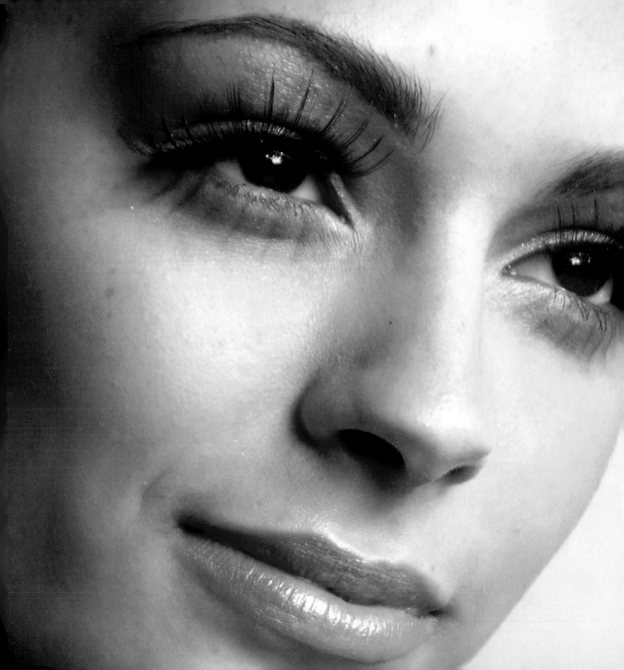

twiggy

Born Lesley Hornby on September 19, 1949, Twiggy was one of the most famous models of her time and "the face" of 1960s swinging London. Her hallmarks were her huge eyes lined with extra-long lashes (both real and painted), as well as her fragile features and super-thin figure—thus her name. She continues to model and act, and is also a great supporter of animal welfare and anti-fur campaigns. Enlarge your eyes as Twiggy did by drawing on lots of false lashes.

INGREDIENTS

eye shadows
iridescent gold
matte orange
matte reddish-brown
matte brown (optional)

other makeup
taupe brow pencil
black mascara
black false eyelashes

brushes
wide eye shadow brush
small eye shadow brush
mini blender brush
eyeliner brush

1. Use **wide brush** to blend gold over upper lid, brow bone, and under eye.

2. Use **small brush** to apply orange to crease, winging it out to create an eyelash shape.

3. Use **mini blender brush** to accentuate crease with reddish-brown.

4. Line lower lid with **brow pencil**.

5. Draw taupe eyelashes under eye with **brow pencil** (or wet a brown eye shadow and apply with an **eyeliner brush**).

6. Use a wet **eyeliner brush** and orange eye shadow to draw orange eyelashes between taupe eyelashes. Repeat above the eye, drawing lashes from the crease and going up.

7. Apply **mascara** and **falsies**.

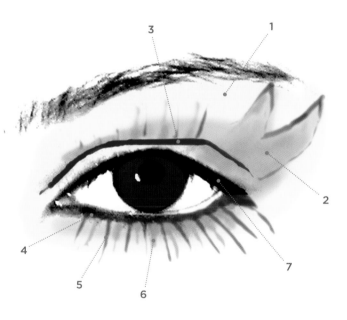

HINT Put colored dots on the ends of the painted lower lashes for a "Pierrot" look.

We finished Marisol's look with reddish-brown cream blush and orange lip gloss.

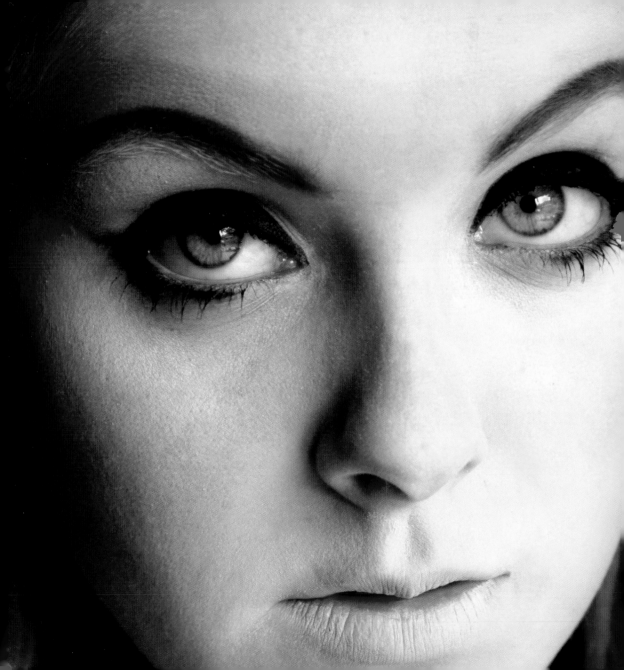

asuka langley soryu

Asuka Langley Soryu is a 14-year-old fictional character from the Japanese anime Neon Genesis Evangelion and the films *Evangelion: Death and Rebirth* and *The End of Evengelion*.

Asuka's proud, strong personality (evocative of a female Samurai) hides and protects a vulnerable and insecure girl, a side we only see in her dreams and thoughts. Her character inspired this unusual, ferocious look.

INGREDIENTS

eye shadows
cream white
cream orange
cream turquoise
semimatte powder turquoise
matte black

other makeup
black pencil eyeliner
brown brow pencil
black mascara

brushes
synthetic concealer brush
small eye shadow brush
mini blender brush

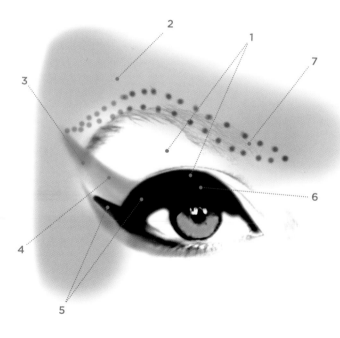

1. Use **fingertips** to blend white over upper lid and brow bone.

2. Use **fingers** to blend orange above brow and around to cheek.

3. Use **synthetic brush** and cream turquoise to make shape on outer brow bone. On opposite eye, dot cream turquoise in the inner corner.

4. Press powder turquoise into turquoise cream with **small brush**.

5. Line lower lid with **eyeliner**, extending past eye. Then apply a thick line to upper lid, blending up and out.

6. Use **mini blender brush** to blend black powder into eyeliner.

7. Strengthen and accentuate brows with **brow pencil**, following dotted guide.

8. Apply lots of **mascara**.

HINT For an even more dramatic look, bring the cream orange shadow down and across the face.

We completed this look on Suzanne with white base on the lips.

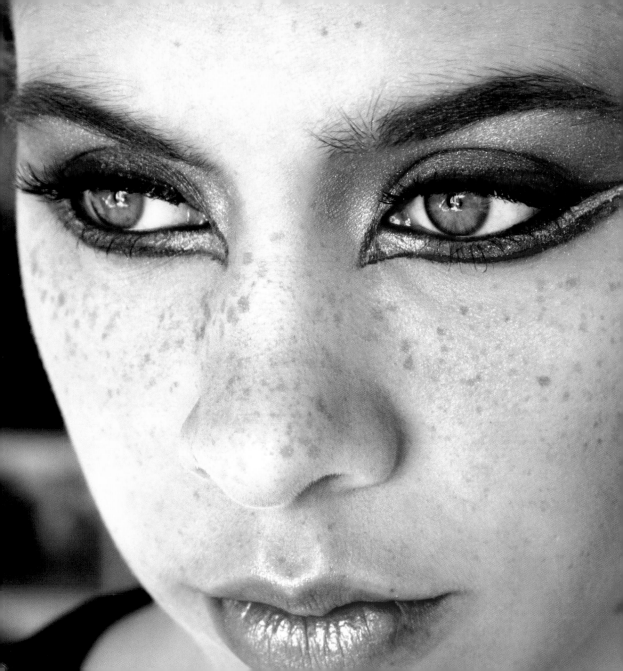

cleopatra

When it comes to legendary drama, few can beat Cleopatra. Born in 69 BC, she became the last queen of Egypt, as her suicide marked the end of the line of Egyptian pharoahs. She is reknowned for her great beauty and her notorious liaisons with Julius Ceasar and Mark Antony, two of the most powerful men of her time. Cleopatra emphasized her opulence with extravagant eye makeup. She would strongly color her lids, lengthen them with eyeliner, and line the inner rims with black kohl.

INGREDIENTS

eye shadows
matte violet
matte deep purple
iridescent aqua
iridescent silver

other makeup
blue cake eyeliner
black pencil eyeliner
black mascara

brushes
large eye shadow brush
small eye shadow brush
eyeliner brush
mini blender brush

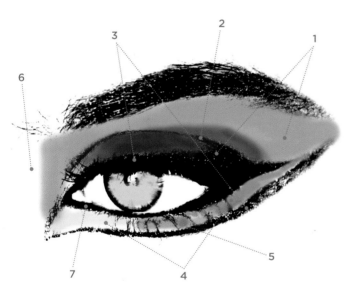

1. Use **large brush** to apply violet over upper lid and brow bone.

2. Use **small brush** to apply purple over upper lid to just past the crease.

3. Use **eyeliner brush** and **blue cake eyeliner** to draw the design around eye, as shown.

4. Use **mini blender brush** to apply aqua inside the design under eye.

5. Use **eyeliner brush** to apply violet inside the design under center of lower eye.

6. Use **small brush** to add silver highlight to inner eye and brow.

7. Line inner rim of lower eye with **black pencil eyeliner**.

8. Apply **mascara**.

HINT To make this look even more opulent, add jewels in place of the aqua in the outer part of the eye.

Daisy's look was finished with a little berry blush and iridescent pink lip gloss.

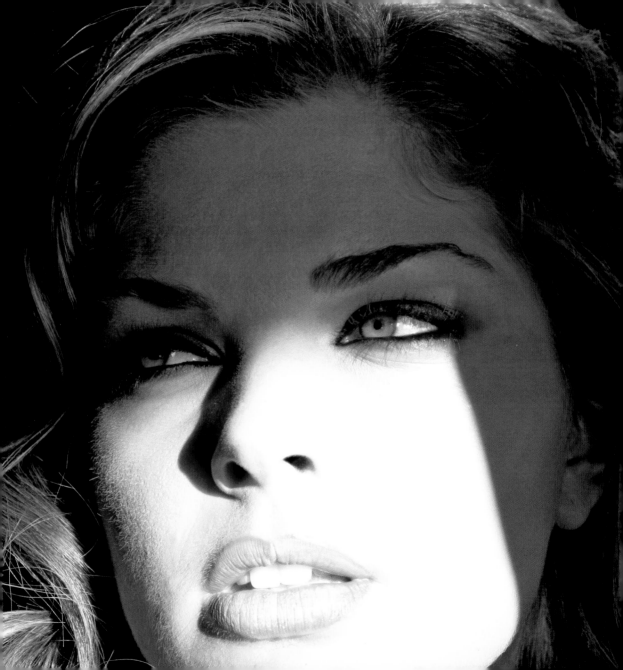

brigitte bardot

Brigitte Bardot, a French actress and model, inspires carefree sensuality. Born September 28, 1934, she became a star in the 1950s and 60s and was famous for her trademark smoky eye and sexy, tousled hair. She later become an animal rights activist, work that she continues to this day. Bardot's famous eye—lined heavily with black—continues to be a favorite with makeup artists and celebrities.

INGREDIENTS

eye shadows
matte dark gray
iridescent pale lilac

other makeup
black pencil eyeliner
black mascara

brushes
small eye shadow brush
eyeliner brush

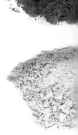

1. Use **small brush** to apply dark gray to upper lid to just past crease and under eye.

2. Use **small brush** to add pale lilac highlight on brow bone.

3. Use **eyeliner** to line inner rim of lower eye.

4. Line upper and lower lash-lines with **eyeliner** and blend the line with **eyeliner brush**.

5. Apply **mascara**.

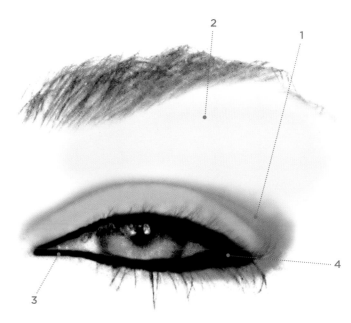

HINT If you have green eyes, try violet eyeliner instead of black. For very dark eyes, try dark blue.

To complete our Bardot look on Nicole, we used neutral blush and nude lipstick covered with yellow gloss.

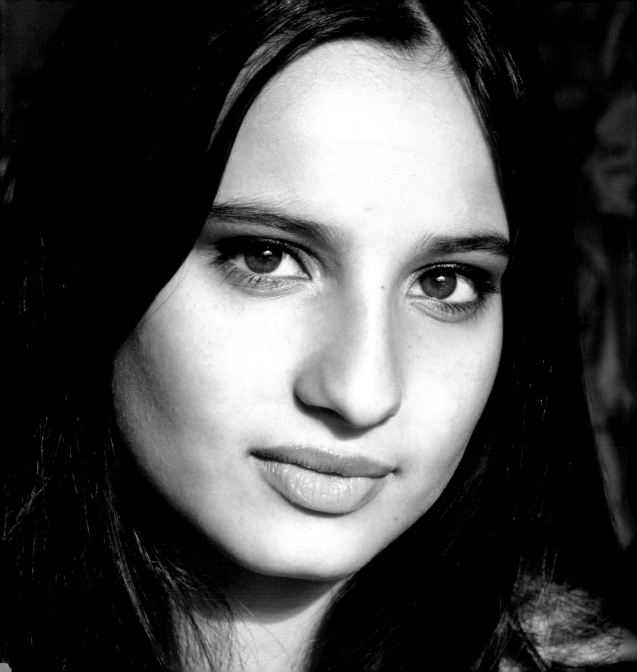

sophia loren

Sophia Loren is a wonderful example of a modern woman who has successfully balanced a full career and family life while keeping her integrity and femininity intact. Born in Italy on September 20, 1934, she became an award-winning film and theater actress. She was a forerunner of celebrity entrepreneurship, with businesses ranging from cookbooks to eyewear, jewelry, and perfume. She is renowned for her exotic beauty, strong almond-shaped eyes, and full lips. Here, we give a modern, colorful twist to her traditional eye makeup while still keeping the exoticism.

INGREDIENTS

eye shadows
iridescent pink
iridescent pale lilac
matte violet

other makeup
navy blue gel eyeliner
black mascara

brushes
wide eye shadow brush
mini blender brush
eyeliner brush

1. Use **wide brush** to blend pink over upper lid and brow bone.

2. Use **mini blender brush** to apply pale lilac to inner corner and under eye.

3. Use **mini blender brush** to blend violet from crease, up and onto brow bone.

4. With **eyeliner brush**, line upper lid with eyeliner. The line should be thick in outer two-thirds of eye and then narrow over pupil and in the inner eye.

5. Finish with **mascara**.

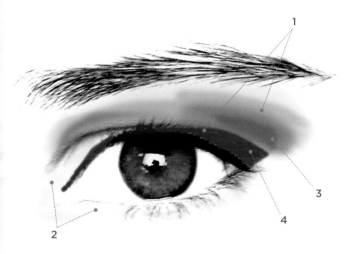

HINT This eyeliner shape is great for anyone with round eyes who wants them to look more almond-shaped.

We kept this look easy to wear on Jaci with soft reddish-brown cream blush and clear lip gloss.

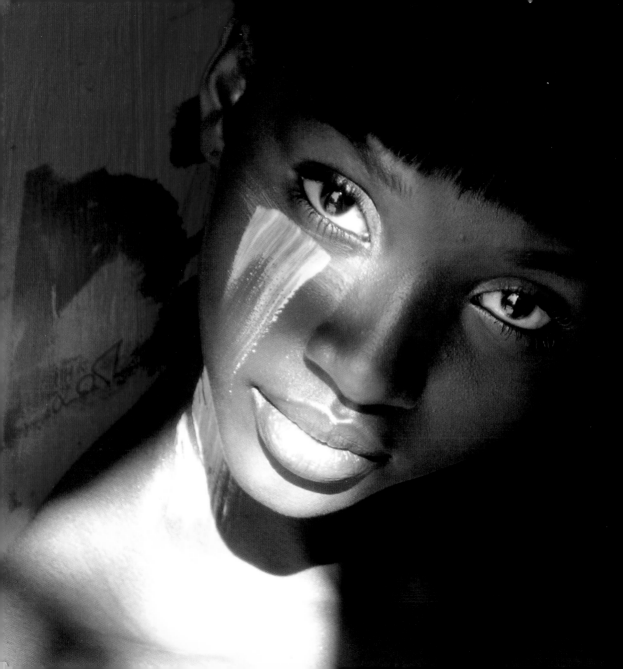

me!

I've been a makeup artist for fashion and beauty photo shoots since 1975, and I generally work with more conventional makeup and looks. But what I am really known for is my creative, freestyle makeup. It's like turning yourself into a total art piece! Use just one or two colors delicately, as shown opposite, or go crazy, like we did below. You don't have to use the Kryolan body paints—although they're fabulous. Try it with any old eye makeup.

INGREDIENTS

eye shadows
Kryolan Aquacolors paint set
(or any old eye makeup)

brushes
paintbrushes

1. Wet a **paintbrush** and load it with iridescent eye shadow or paint from the Kryolan set. Swipe it near your eyes or over your lids and brows.

2. Rub **clear lip gloss** on your cheeks and then crumble up your paints or old matte shadows and press them into the gloss.

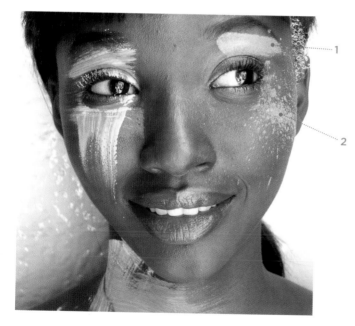

HINT Your look doesn't have to be as obvious as the ones shown here—it can be as simple as a dot of gloss on your lids with crumbled powder pressed into it with your fingertip. Just let the idea inspire you and experiment—it's only makeup, after all!

Rose's freestyle makeup was built over her Bright Eyes look on page 115.

makeup directory

You can use any makeup brands to create the looks in this book—just use the palettes provided to find the right shades. But if you want to know *exactly* what was used for each look, here is a list of the colors from my own line of makeup, available at Linda Mason's The Art of Beauty in New York City, or online at www.lindamason.com or www.daisym.com.

everyday

Sparkle: Antique and Celebration eye shadows; Country lip gloss

Polished: Peach Sunrise and Mushroom eye shadows; Gin cream blush; Opera lip gloss

Posh: Mediterranean, Brown Earth, and Gold Bar eye shadows; Coral matte blush; Coral lip color and Fire lip gloss

Earth Angel: Lilac, Mist, and Peach Sunrise eye shadows; Coral matte blush; Opera lip gloss

Casual: Peach Sunrise and Red Earth eye shadows; Earth cake eyeliner; Classical lip gloss

Coquette: Mushroom and Lilac Cloud eye shadows; Black Russian cream blush; Folk lip gloss

Golden: Ivory, Mustard, and Sacrifice eye shadows; Black Russian cream blush; Fire lip gloss

Smooth: Peach Sunrise and Red Earth eye shadows; Black Russian cream blush; Brick lip color

Soulful: Stone and Storm eye shadows; Black Russian cream blush; Coral lip color

Lucky: Glimmer Green, Kiwi, and Evergreen eye shadows; Gin cream blush; Orange lip color and Fire lip gloss

Punky: Loose Aqua Impact, Dulcinea, and Loose Pink Impact eye shadows; Ebony cake eyeliner; Sugar Plum blush; Folk lip gloss

flirtatious

Dazzle: Kingfisher and Gold Bar eye shadows; Gin cream blush; Coral lip color

Bronze Shimmer: Lilac Cloud and Mushroom eye shadows; Copper gel eyeliner; Black Russian cream blush; Brown lip color

Mystery: Fuchsia Jewel and Silver Platinum eye shadows; Black Russian cream blush; Folk lip gloss

Eye Contact: Cat's Eye, Green Jewel, and Forest Bed eye shadows; Coral matte blush; Opera lip gloss

Dreamy: Seafoam (cream), Ocean Gold, and Silver Bullet eye shadows; Black Russian cream blush; Classical lip gloss

Glow: Gold Bar and Coal eye shadows; Ebony pencil eyeliner; Black Russian cream blush; Fire lip gloss

Fresh: Green Foam, Mist, and Purple eye shadows; Flash blush; Babe lipstick

Galaxy Girl: Seafoam (semimatte), Mist, and Khaki eye shadows; Jazz lip gloss

Think Pink: Shell, Fuchsia, Pearl, and Ocean eye shadows; Rock lip gloss

Spring Fling: Shell and Kingfisher eye shadows; Water cake eyeliner; Black Russian cream blush; Opera lip gloss

Colorful: Loose Orange Impact, Loose Pink Impact, Loose Violet Impact, and Dulcinea eye shadows; Martini cream blush; Classical lip gloss

funky

Neon: Loose Impact Orange, Loose Impact Yellow, Loose Impact Lime, and Loose Impact Pink eye shadows; Hot Pink lipstick

Electric: Hot Pink, Amethyst, Sand, and Emerald eye shadows; Gin cream blush; Fuchsia Impact lip color

Urban Poet: Rose Petal, Pink Heaven, Turquoise (semimatte), and Sand eye shadows; Hot Pink lip color

Moulin Rouge: Flame, Ocean Gold, and Sand eye shadows; Ebony pencil eyeliner; Black Russian cream blush; Jazz lip gloss

Firestarter: Rose Red and Pink Sapphire eye shadows; Red Fire pencil eyeliner; Coral matte blush; Folk lip gloss

Playful: Shell, Silver Bullet, Mist, and Aqua Tint eye shadows; Truth blush; Jazz lip gloss

Beatnik: Orange and Evergreen eye shadows; Fire lip gloss; Pearl lip color

Bejeweled: Kiwi, Green Jewel, Glimmer, and Purple Jewel eye shadows; Black Russian cream blush; Coral lip color and Folk lip gloss

Odyssey: White and Coal eye shadows; Ebony pencil eyeliner; Flash blush; Pink lip color

Abstraction: Orange, Evergreen, Silver Bullet, and Yellow Rose eye shadows; Water cake eyeliner; Fire lip gloss

Vanity: Aqua, Ocean, and Aquafoam eye shadows; Water cake eyeliner; Rose matte blush; Opera lip gloss

Mardi Gras: Seafoam (cream), Olive You, Navy, Amethyst, and Aqua eye shadows; Water cake eyeliner; Scarlett lipstick

glamorous

Bright Eyes: Ocean and Ocean Foam eye shadows; Ebony pencil eyeliner; Martini cream blush; Tallulah lipstick

Oomph: Mushroom, Brown Earth, Storm, Dark Mink, and Coal eye shadows; Ebony pencil eyeliner; Driftwood blush; Nude lip color and Fire lip gloss

Blue Mood: Aqua Foam, Aqua, and Turquoise (semi-matte) eye shadows; Hunter pencil eyeliner; Coral matte blush; Shy lip gel and Muted Pink lip color

Exotic: Tarnish, Pure Gold, and Pacific eye shadows; Martini cream blush; Punk lip gloss

Celestial: Navy, Coal, and Pearl eye shadows; Ebony pencil eyeliner; Gin cream blush; Jazz lip gloss

Knockout: Lilac Cloud, Storm, and Coal eye shadows; Ebony pencil eyeliner; Emperor blush; Nude lip color

Zingara: Glimmer Green, Turquoise (semimatte), and Witchcraft eye shadows; Ebony pencil eyeliner; Black Russian cream blush; Opera lip gloss

Royal: Lilac, Mist, Purple, and Lilac Cloud eye shadows; Ebony pencil eyeliner; Berry matte blush; Babe lipstick

Warrior: Sand, Khaki, Red Earth, and Coal eye shadows; Ebony pencil eyeliner; Emperor blush; Scarlett lipstick

X Factor: Glimmer, Olive You, and Coal eye shadows; Ebony pencil eyeliner; Latin lip gloss

Midnight: Navy, Coal, and Seafoam (semimatte) eye shadows; Ebony pencil eyeliner; Gin cream blush; Jazz lip gloss

inspired

Audrey Hepburn: Khaki and Snow White eye shadows; Black cake eyeliner; Coral matte blush; Beth lipstick

Mata Hari: Kiwi, Mediterranean, and Green Foam eye shadows; Gin cream blush; Jazz lip gloss

Marilyn Monroe: Snow White and Mushroom eye shadows; Flush blush; Audrey lipstick

Sunset: Nikiya Mieral and Fuchsia Impact eye shadows; Jane lipstick

Twiggy: Gold Bar, Orange, and Red Earth eye shadows; Natural Taupe brow pencil; Black Russian cream blush; Latin lip gloss

Asuka Langley Soryu: White, Ginger, Turquoise (cream), Turquoise (semimatte), and Coal eye shadows; Ebony pencil eyeliner; Brunette brow pencil

Cleopatra: Mist, Purple, Aqua, and Silver Platinum eye shadows; Water cake eyeliner; Ebony pencil eyeliner; Berry matte blush; Jazz lip gloss

Brigitte Bardot: Storm and Lilac Cloud eye shadows; Ebony pencil eyeliner; Driftwood matte blush; Nude lip color and Fire lip gloss

Sophia Loren: Shell, Lilac Cloud, and Mist eye shadows; Scuba gel eyeliner; Black Russian cream blush; Folk lip gloss

Linda Mason: Kryolan Aquacolors paint set

index